4 steps to
lower
cholesterol

4 steps to *lower* cholesterol

The practical guide to a healthy heart

LINDA MAIN AND BALDEESH RAI

Vermilion
LONDON

1 3 5 7 9 10 8 6 4 2

Vermilion, an imprint of Ebury Publishing,
20 Vauxhall Bridge Road,
London SW1V 2SA

Vermilion is part of the Penguin Random House group of companies
whose addresses can be found at global.penguinrandomhouse.com

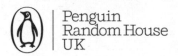

Copyright © Linda Main and Baldeesh Rai 2015

Linda Main and Baldeesh Rai have asserted their right to be
identified as the authors of this Work in accordance with the
Copyright, Designs and Patents Act 1988

First published by Vermilion in 2015

www.eburypublishing.co.uk

A CIP catalogue record for this book is available from the British Library

ISBN 9781785040177

Printed and bound in Great Britain by Clays Ltd, St Ives PLC

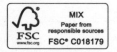

Penguin Random House is committed to a
sustainable future for our business, our readers
and our planet. This book is made from Forest
Stewardship Council® certified paper.

Contents

Foreword

Welcome to *4 Steps to Lower Cholesterol*, a wise purchase if you are looking to know all about cholesterol – including how to lower it and improve your heart health.

Over the years there has been much confusion and controversy about what to eat to maintain a healthy heart, and it's no wonder that many of us are still unsure of what we should and shouldn't eat. Sadly, sometimes the message about what to eat gets over-simplified and this has been the issue for cholesterol.

Cholesterol is an important risk factor for heart disease and it is not just the old or the overweight who are at risk. Many young people also have high cholesterol and are completely unaware of it until a routine test or a family member alerts them to the fact that they may have inherited it.

This book is suitable for anyone looking to improve their cholesterol, whether it has been raised through lifestyle factors or is an inherited condition.

In this book, Baldeesh and Linda dispel the myths surrounding cholesterol. Both Linda and Baldeesh are registered dietitians with many years of experience dealing with queries regarding cholesterol management. With their help, you will be able to discover cholesterol-busting foods and eating patterns that help to lower cholesterol, for use either alone or alongside medications such as statins.

I hope you make the best use of this book, including the fabulous recipes (all very easy to follow, inexpensive and based on readily available ingredients) and the many resources, tools and tips, each one designed to make your life easier by providing the necessary help for you to make sustainable small changes that add up to a healthier heart.

Finally thank you for purchasing this book. A small contribution from each sale comes directly to HEART UK and we make good use of this to maintain and develop our activities. HEART UK – The Cholesterol Charity is the only UK charity dedicated to people with high cholesterol. Through our website, resources and helpline we aim to support, educate, guide and empower families to make changes to their diet and lifestyle and to understand the facts behind the research and media headlines.

If you wish to know more about HEART UK, the work we do and how you might get involved, why not visit us at www.heartuk.org.uk.

Good luck
Jules Payne
Chief Executive
HEART UK – The Cholesterol Charity

Introduction

This book was written to support anyone struggling or concerned about the long-term effects of living with raised cholesterol. Does this sound like you? Perhaps you have been trying to manage your cholesterol for years but have been confused by mixed messages. Or you may have tried to make changes but haven't been able to stick to them. Or perhaps you've only just been diagnosed and don't know where to start. Rest assured, there really are simple ways to improve your cholesterol and keep your heart healthier and this book will show you how.

Balancing your diet when you have high cholesterol can be challenging but it's far from impossible. Our own experiences with people diagnosed with raised cholesterol show that provided you receive practical, clear and realistic advice you can become your own expert in managing your cholesterol. Enabling you to achieve this success is what this book is all about.

We have split the book into two parts. The first part helps to demystify cholesterol and enables you to understand the role it plays in cardiovascular (heart and circulatory) disease, as well as empowering you to have a frank and open discussion with your doctor.

Few books tackle the main reasons of why cholesterol is raised, so we aim to highlight how genetics as well as lifestyle play a key role. We also clarify the role of triglycerides, another blood fat linked to cardiovascular disease. The information contained in the book is aimed both at people with inherited forms of high cholesterol and those diagnosed with raised cholesterol as a result of a health MOT or routine screening.

The second part of the book offers you a practical, effective and easy-to-stick-to approach to lowering your cholesterol. It will explain clearly what you can do and how to do it – offering simple advice in a step-by-step approach. We also explain the role of medicines used in cholesterol reduction and set the record straight on statins, the most commonly used cholesterol-lowering drug.

The book contains lots of practical tools including healthy recipes, a helpful shopping list, easy food swaps and some real-life case studies to illustrate the results that can be achieved.

We wish you the very best on your journey with us; you might find it helpful to keep a record of the changes you make so that you can reflect back in the next few weeks just how far you have actually come.

PART 1

CHAPTER 1

Understanding cholesterol

Firstly things first: just what is cholesterol exactly? Cholesterol is a type of fat that is found in our blood and in every single cell in our body. In the media, cholesterol is often described as harmful and most headlines focus on the relationship between high levels of cholesterol in the blood and the increased risk of heart disease. However, cholesterol also has a vital role to play in maintaining the healthy functioning of our bodies. Cholesterol only becomes a problem if we have too much of it.

Our increasingly unhealthy lifestyles and the fact that most of us are living longer, means that many more people today are living with unhealthy levels of cholesterol. And being a significant risk factor for heart disease, this means it is putting many of us at greater risk of a heart attack. According to the World Health Organisation, raised blood cholesterol is one of the top ten causes of death throughout the world.

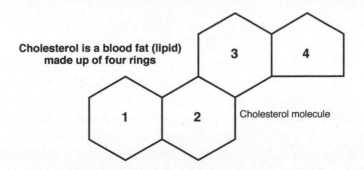

Cholesterol is a blood fat (lipid) made up of four rings

Cholesterol molecule

How long have we been aware of cholesterol?

The role of cholesterol and other blood fats in health and disease has been the subject of extensive research since the nineteenth century. Cholesterol itself was first described as early as 1816, and by the 1830s researchers had identified the unique way that cholesterol is transported around the body. By 1845 cholesterol was known to be a component in the fatty plaques that block arteries.

This early research continued throughout the early twentieth century and by 1913 Anitschow, a Russian pathologist, established through observing changes in the arteries of rabbits that cholesterol was key to the development of fatty plaques inside the walls of critical blood vessels, such as the coronary arteries, which ultimately leads to heart disease.

Since then researchers and doctors have begun to unravel the complex biological role that cholesterol and other related blood fats play in the body, including the role of diet and lifestyle in helping to manage cholesterol levels.

Several drug types have been developed to help lower cholesterol and among these are statins, easily the most powerful and effective of all these medicines. The first statin was made available to treat high cholesterol (sometimes known as hyperlipidaemia, dyslipidaemia or hypercholesterolaemia) in 1987. Since then this category of drugs has expanded so that there are five statins available to patients in the UK, at varying doses, and the number of people taking them has grown exponentially. This dramatic increase in statin usage is partly responsible for the reduction in heart disease seen in the UK in more recent years.

The prevention of heart disease and stroke remain very close to the top of the UK's health priorities, and encouraging people to live a healthy lifestyle is key to this. For those living with heart disease or stroke, or at increased risk of developing them, new and evolving research is essential to help us to develop new drug and treatment therapies which can be used alongside of, or in some cases instead of, statins.

Where does cholesterol come from?

Cholesterol comes from two sources:

- We make it ourselves (synthesised or endogenous cholesterol)
- We get it from food (dietary or exogenous cholesterol).

Synthesised (endogenous) cholesterol

The amount of cholesterol our bodies make is dependent upon how much we consume, but we have the ability to make most, or all of, our cholesterol. Typically we need about 1 g of cholesterol from our food and from synthesis everyday.

Every cell in the body has the ability to make cholesterol; however, most is produced in the liver. Other organs that make a significant amount of cholesterol include the intestines, adrenal glands and reproductive organs.

As you read through the book you will notice that we mention lipids, so it might be helpful if we define them now. 'Lipid' is another word for fat, but it is only usually used for fats that are inside the body. So cholesterol in food is a fat, but cholesterol in the blood is a lipid.

Dietary (exogenous) cholesterol

By comparison with other fats, dietary cholesterol is poorly absorbed. The amount of cholesterol you absorb can vary significantly from person to person because it can be influenced by the genes you inherit from your parents. Typically we eat between 100 and 400 mg of cholesterol per day. Cholesterol is only found in animal products.

There is no doubt that dietary cholesterol can raise blood cholesterol levels but the effect seems to be modest when compared to that of saturated fats in the diet. Why? It appears that the body tries to compensate for any increase in the absorption of dietary cholesterol. It does this by reducing cholesterol synthesis. This is why dietary advice for most people does not include the need to restrict cholesterol intake. Occasionally it is necessary to restrict organ meats like liver and kidney, which are very rich in cholesterol.

As we will learn in chapter 2, saturated fat has a much more potent effect in increasing cholesterol levels and is of greater public health concern. Happily, by restricting saturated fat intake, we also restrict cholesterol intake as they are found in similar foods, for example, full-fat dairy products, meat and meat products. However, egg yolks, shellfish and organ meats, such as liver and kidney, all contain a lot of cholesterol, but are generally lower in saturated fat.

Why do we need cholesterol?

Cholesterol plays a vital role in the day-to-day functioning of our bodies. Without cholesterol we simply could not survive. It has two main roles: structural and regulatory. One of its most vital functions is the role it plays in the growth and repair of cells. Every single cell in the body contains cholesterol. Together with other fats and proteins, cholesterol is jointly responsible for the complex outer structure of each cell, which we call the cell membrane. A mixture of fatty components (cholesterol, phospholipids and fatty acids) are arranged in layers to form the cell membrane. Their water-loving (hydrophilic) ends face outwards from the cell and also in towards the inner cellular space. Their fat-loving (hydrophobic) ends face inwards towards the centre of the membrane. This structure forms a very effective 'watertight' barrier. Along the surface of the cell membrane are complex proteins or 'carriers'. The function of these carriers is to actively allow nutrients in and out of the cell and allow waste to be removed from the cell.

The structure of cell membranes

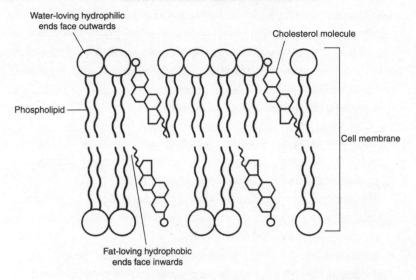

Water-loving hydrophilic ends face outwards

Cholesterol molecule

Phospholipid

Cell membrane

Fat-loving hydrophobic ends face inwards

Cholesterol is also needed to make several hormones, each of which is needed to control one of more key regulatory functions in the body. For example, cholesterol forms the basic building block needed for the production of vitamin D. Part of this process requires cholesterol (in the form of 7–dehydrocholesterol) to accumulate in the skin where it is converted to a vitamin D precursor using UV sunlight. This pre-vitamin is then further converted to the active form of vitamin D in the liver and kidneys.

Vitamin D is needed for the absorption of calcium from our diet and to control the amount of calcium present in bone, teeth and the blood. It is believed that vitamin D may also have a role in protecting our hearts and circulatory systems.

In reality, skin synthesis of vitamin D from cholesterol is responsible for most of our vitamin D. Diet can provide some, but very few foods are rich in vitamin D and even fewer in winter due to seasonal variation. In the UK our dietary intake of vitamin D is poor at best, and in some people may be very poor.

For young children, pregnant and breastfeeding women, older people or where an individual's skin is routinely covered, highly pigmented or not exposed to sunlight, skin synthesis of vitamin D may not be enough on its own. So for these groups it is generally agreed that there is a need for a supplemental form of vitamin D.

Cholesterol is also essential to make:

- **Cortisol** – a hormone produced by the adrenal glands. We have two adrenal glands which sit on top of each of our kidneys. Cortisol regulates the body's response to stress.
- **Aldosterone** – a hormone whose main function is to ensure that the levels of electrolytes (sodium, chloride and potassium) are carefully controlled in the body.
- **Testosterone**, which is produced by the male testes and is responsible for male sexual characteristics and sperm production.
- **Progesterone**, which is produced by the female ovaries, and is responsible for female sexual characteristics.

Bile

Bile salts help to ensure our digestive system works properly. Bile is made in the liver from the breakdown of cholesterol and together with some cholesterol passes into the gut, via the bile duct, in response to eating a meal. The role of bile in digestion is to help emulsify dietary fat. This emulsification breaks the fat down into tiny microscopic droplets, with a very large surface area, which allows the fat to mix with digestive enzymes.

Lower down the gut these cholesterol-rich bile salts pass into the colon, or large intestine. Surplus cholesterol is usually excreted in this way but not all is lost as large percentages of both bile and cholesterol are reabsorbed and recycled. We refer to this recycling of bile and cholesterol in chapter 2.

Occasionally, cholesterol that collects in the bile duct can start to crystallise to form one or more gallstones. Over time these stones can become quite large and painful, requiring removal by keyhole surgery. If not removed these stones will continue to grow and may eventually block the bile duct completely, resulting in fatty stools (as the fat is not properly digested and absorbed), inflamed bile ducts and potentially causing damage to the liver.

The cholesterol transport system

Here comes the scientific bit. Don't be tempted to skip this as understanding the cholesterol transport system is fundamental to:

- Understanding any tests or blood results you have
- Helping you understand more about your condition
- Understanding how dietary change or medication can work for you.

First of all it is important to understand that the liver is the central organ for handling cholesterol and other blood lipids. It makes and prepares cholesterol for transport to all the other organs.

We have all seen how fat floats on top of water and when the two are mixed together they rapidly separate on standing. It is the same with cholesterol and blood. Because cholesterol is a lipid it cannot travel around the body loose because it can't dissolve in the blood. Instead, along with other blood lipids, it has its own transport system, which enables it to be carried around the body. Cholesterol is carried in special parcels, which act like taxis in the body. There are lots of these special taxis and they travel in the blood to every part of the body. Each taxi is a very small particle and is called a lipoprotein.

As their name implies – lipo (lipid) protein (protein) – these taxis are made up of a number of blood lipids:

- Cholesterol
- Triglycerides (another type of blood lipid)
- Phospholipids.

and one or more specialised proteins called apolipoproteins (sometimes shortened to apoproteins or apos).

Similar to the role of bile in the gastrointestinal tract, phospholipids act as detergents to help emulsify fats. The proteins are needed to help to keep the taxis stable.

There are four main types of special taxis or lipoproteins, all of which have slightly different functions and which get their names from their relative density. Density is a measure of their weight, their contents and how compact they are. The lower the density of the lipoprotein, the greater the amount of lipid contained within it.

The four main types of lipoproteins and their functions

Lipoprotein	Main function
Chylomicrons (the least dense type of cholesterol transport molecules)	Transports triglycerides and free fatty acids from the intestines to tissues where they will be used or stored as fuel
VLDL (very low-density lipoprotein)	Transport excess triglycerides and free fatty acids from the liver to adipose tissue (fat storage tissue) and muscle
LDL (low-density lipoproteins)	The main carrier of cholesterol from the liver to tissues with excess returning to the liver
HDL (high-density lipoproteins)	Transport surplus cholesterol from tissues back to the liver for processing

The two lipoproteins that are most often referred to are low-density lipoprotein (LDL) and high-density lipoproteins (HDL).

Low-density lipoprotein (LDL) is often called the carrier of bad cholesterol. LDLs are cholesterol-rich particles. About 70 per cent of the cholesterol in the blood is carried on these LDL taxis. Their main role is to transport cholesterol, which is packaged up in the liver and sent to the tissues, where it is used for growth, repair and hormone production.

The LDL taxi

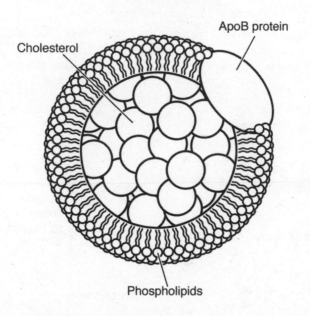

LDL cholesterol is taken into cells through special transport 'portholes' using a form of 'lock-and-key' mechanism. To work, the mechanism needs two parts. Each porthole, on the surface of the cell, forms the lock. It consists of a cellular pit made of protein – and is called an LDL receptor. The LDL taxis have a special protein on their surface called apolipoprotein B (or apoB for short). This protein forms the key and becomes attached to the lock in the cell membrane. It is this lock-and-key mechanism that opens the LDL receptor and lets the LDL taxi into the cell. Here its contents are broken down into free cholesterol and amino acids. Most of each cell's cholesterol needs are met in this way.

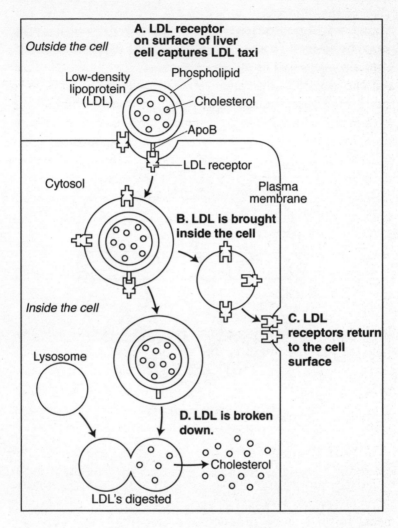

In some people not all of the LDL receptors work properly. If this is the case the levels of LDL cholesterol in the blood are usually high, sometimes two, three or even four times the normal levels. This general understanding of how LDL receptors work will also help you to understand how statins work when we come to chapter 9.

The term 'LDL cholesterol' refers to the cholesterol carried in the LDL taxi.

High-density lipoproteins (HDL) are often called the carrier of good cholesterol. These particles are formed mainly in the liver. They are composed of 50 per cent protein, with phospholipid and cholesterol as the remainder. The role of the HDL is to transport excess cholesterol from the tissues (including the arterial wall) to the liver for recycling and excretion. HDL is famously known for its protective role against cardiovascular disease. Its protective properties include anti-inflammatory and antioxidant activity, which help it protect the artery wall against LDL cholesterol and may help to slow the disease process, which normally leads to the furring up of blood vessels which in turn lead to cardiovascular disease.

The term 'HDL cholesterol' refers to the cholesterol carried in the HDL taxi.

Triglyceride is a special name given to fats and describes how they are found in nature. 'Tri' means three, and 'glyceride' comes from glycerol, a three-carbon molecule. Triglycerides are essentially made from one molecule of glycerol, which is attached to three fatty acids, one to each carbon. These fatty acids could be the same or different. They could all be saturated or unsaturated or a mixture. It might help to imagine a triglyceride as a tuning fork with the glycerol being the short bit in the middle and the two prongs and handle being the three fatty acids. Triglycerides occur naturally in foods such as meat, full-fat dairy produce and cooking oils. They are absorbed in the intestines and then transported in the blood to the tissues where they are either stored as fat or used to provide energy.

Trigylcerides are also made in the liver. When more calories are consumed than our bodies require, the liver forms triglycerides from this excess energy. Any surplus triglycerides are then transported to a specialised type of tissue called adipose where they are stored until needed.

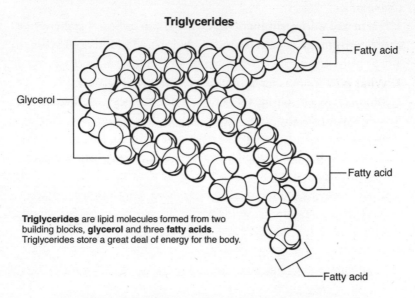

Triglycerides

Glycerol

Fatty acid

Fatty acid

Fatty acid

Triglycerides are lipid molecules formed from two building blocks, **glycerol** and three **fatty acids**. Triglycerides store a great deal of energy for the body.

Simplified Illustration of a Triglyceride and a Phospholipid

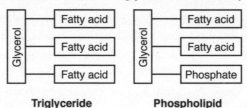

Triglyceride

Phospholipid

Chylomicrons and VLDLs are the two triglyceride-rich taxis. Chylomicrons carry triglycerides from the intestines to the liver and VLDLs carry triglycerides from the liver to the tissues where they are either stored or used for energy.

Blood tests and results

In most cases there are no outward signs or symptoms that can tell you what your cholesterol level might be. The only definitive way to find out your cholesterol level is to have a cholesterol test. You can arrange a simple cholesterol test at your doctor's surgery and tests are also available at many high-street pharmacies.

Here are some simple questions to ask when having your cholesterol tested:

1. What is being measured, or what results will I receive?

You may receive information on one or all of the following:

- Total cholesterol – the total amount of cholesterol in the blood
- LDL cholesterol – the amount of cholesterol carried on the LDL taxi in the blood
- HDL cholesterol – the amount of cholesterol carried on the HDL taxi in the blood
- Triglycerides – the total amount of triglycerides in the blood
- Total cholesterol to HDL ratio – the amount of total cholesterol divided by HDL cholesterol.

2. Do I need to fast overnight?

- Fasting is only usually necessary if your blood test is designed to measure triglycerides or if your doctor is trying to make a diagnosis. If you are having a fasting test then avoid eating and have only water for 12 hours before the test. It is less disruptive if you arrange this test early in the morning as you will have fasted overnight.
- The test measures how well your body is clearing triglycerides out of the blood. After fasting for 12 hours your triglyceride levels should be very low.
- Blood levels of cholesterol are not greatly affected by a recent meal but it's wise to stick to your normal dietary routine rather than have something that is unusually high in fat or sugar before any blood test.

3. How is my blood taken?

- It is possible to do a cholesterol test from a finger-prick sample of blood these days. We call this a capillary sample as it comes from a capillary, a tiny blood vessel, in your finger. Some doctors prefer to take a larger blood sample from a vein for diagnostic purposes.

4. How long will it take to get a result?

- Some tests can give you an instant reading while others may take up to a week because the blood has to be sent away to a laboratory.

5. Will my overall cardiovascular risk be explained?

- Doctors, practice nurses and high-street pharmacists will often calculate your overall cardiovascular risk as part of a general health check. This is only useful if you have not already been diagnosed with a heart or circulatory condition. If you already have a diagnosis then ask your doctor about your risk when you next have a routine check-up.

There are two main ways of having your cholesterol tested:

The Gold Standard: full-fasting lipid profile (method 1)

This is usually used for diagnostic or research purposes. If you are having this kind of test you will be asked to fast for a 12–hour period. A doctor, nurse or a phlebotomist, a specialist trained to take blood samples, will take a sample of blood from a vein, usually in your arm, and will send this to an accredited laboratory for analysis. Because your doctor has requested that all your blood lipids are determined, this is known as a full lipid profile. It includes measurements of total cholesterol (TC), HDL cholesterol (HDL), and triglycerides (TG). LDL cholesterol (LDL) is not measured but is calculated from the levels of other blood fats. Your total cholesterol to HDL-cholesterol ratio (TC:HDL) will also be calculated.

Point-of-care or screening test (method 2)

This is a simple test which can be carried out in minutes and can be performed either fasting or non-fasting. A calibrated point-of-care testing device is used. A small but carefully measured quantity of blood is taken, usually from a finger. The blood is placed on a cassette or a special strip that is then inserted into the point-of-care meter. The result is available within a few minutes. The lipoproteins and lipids that are measured depend upon the cassette or strip that is used and can vary from a simple total cholesterol to a full lipid profile. This kind of test is more likely to be used for screening purposes, although the low cost per use and the instant feed-back means they are becoming more widely available in GP surgeries.

Ongoing cholesterol monitoring

If you are found to have a level of cholesterol that needs treatment, your doctor should continue to measure your cholesterol at least once a year. This monitoring process can be done using either a capillary (finger-prick) sample or by sending a larger venous sample for laboratory analysis.

In 2014 a change to the routine way in which cholesterol blood samples are collected was suggested. Once these changes are implemented it will be unnecessary in most cases to fast before a cholesterol test. There will be some exceptions though, so if unclear be sure to ask your doctor or health professional before your appointment.

What should your results be?

In the UK, cholesterol and triglycerides are usually measured in millimoles per litre (mmol/l) but in some countries they are measured in milligrams per decilitre (mg/dl). You can convert from one to another using a simple conversion factor.

To convert cholesterol levels:

Cholesterol mg/dl (Total, LDL and HDL) = mmol/l × 38.6
Cholesterol mmol/l (Total, LDL and HDL) = mg/dl ÷ 38.6

To covert triglyceride levels:

Triglyceride mg/dl = mmol/l × 88.5
Triglyceride mmol/l = mg/dl ÷ 88.5

Examples:

A cholesterol of 5 mmol/l = 193 mg/dl (5 × 38.6)
A triglyceride of 2 mmol/l = 177 mg/dl (2 × 88.5)
A cholesterol of 250 mg/dl = 6.49 mmol/l (250 ÷ 38.5)
A triglyceride of 400 mg/dl = 4.52 mmol/l (400 ÷ 88.5)

We have expressed our recommendations for cholesterol levels in millimoles per litre, as this is the main way of reporting and recording cholesterol in the UK.

It is not possible to give a definitive recommendation for cholesterol levels on which all experts agree. In part, this is because most doctors believe the lower the amount of LDL cholesterol in the blood the better, and partly because cardiovascular disease is caused by multiple factors. Treatment targets are usually agreed upon in consultation with patients and based upon the level of cholesterol at diagnosis and the overall risk to the patient.

The guidelines we provide below have been split into those for healthy adults and those for people who are already considered at higher risk of cardiovascular disease. If you have already been made aware that you are at higher risk of cardiovascular disease then you should speak to your doctor about how far you should lower your cholesterol level. People who are considered to be at higher risk of cardiovascular disease include those with:

- Established coronary heart disease (CHD)
- Other major heart and circulatory conditions
- People with hypertension, significantly raised blood lipids, diabetes, family history of premature CHD, or a combination of these risk factors, which puts them at high risk of heart disease.

	Recommendations for healthy adults	Recommendations for high risk*
Total cholesterol	5 mmol/l or less	
LDL cholesterol	3 mmol/l or less	1.8 mmol/l or less
Non-HDL cholesterol		2.5 mmol/l or less
HDL cholesterol	Men above 1.0 mmol/l Women above 1.2 mmol/l	Men above 1.0 mmol/l Women above 1.2 mmol/l
Fasting triglycerides	Below 1.7 mmol/l	Below 1.7 mmol/l
TC:HDL Ratio	Less than 5	The lower the better

*Doctors often set individual targets for people at high risk

Non-HDL cholesterol is a newer measure of cholesterol and represents the total amount of cholesterol in the blood minus any cholesterol carried on the HDL taxi.

Know your numbers

In order to understand the risk that cholesterol poses to your health it is important to know your results and understand them. It's often best to arrange to see or telephone your GP or practice nurse and ask them to explain the results to you. Don't be afraid to ask questions if your doctor just says your results are normal or nothing to worry about. Be sure to ask what was measured, what the results are, and what this means for your health.

Sometimes the receptionist at the surgery is able to give you your cholesterol results. While this might be helpful, remember they are not a healthcare professional. They may only offer you the total cholesterol result, rather than the full profile of lipids that were measured, and it is very unlikely that they can interpret them for you.

Whatever your results, keep a note of them and the date they were measured. Whenever your cholesterol is checked you should always have a measure of the quality of your cholesterol, such as the amount of HDL cholesterol, LDL cholesterol or non-HDL cholesterol. You can use these results to help track how your results change in the future, but remember always to compare like with like. For example you should not compare a fasting with a non-fasting test result.

Understanding your results

I only know my total cholesterol – is that enough?

While your total cholesterol level is important to know, it is only a measure of the amount of cholesterol in your blood. It does not measure the quality of the cholesterol and tells you very little about your risk of developing cardiovascular disease.

As a minimum you should know a little about both the **quantity** and the **quality** of the cholesterol in your blood. Use your total cholesterol level to give you the amount of cholesterol in your blood and your HDL cholesterol, non-HDL cholesterol or LDL cholesterol to give you a measure of the quality of cholesterol.

What is the TC:HDL ratio?

This is also a measure of the quality of cholesterol in your blood. To determine this you need your total cholesterol and your HDL cholesterol. Then divide the total cholesterol value by the HDL-cholesterol value to get the ratio. The TC:HDL ratio is normally used to help predict heart disease risk.

Ratios above 6 mmol/l indicate a higher risk of heart disease. Ideally your ratio should be below 5.

By now your should have a better understanding of what cholesterol is and its vital role in our body. If you are still unclear, it might be worth reading some of the sections of this chapter again as they form the foundation of some of the key steps in our action plan in chapters 6–9. The way in which cholesterol is transported around the body is fundamental to understanding exactly how statins and some food types help to lower cholesterol and whether their effects are additive. And by understanding exactly how cholesterol is measured and what your results mean we hope this chapter will have empowered you to have a more meaningful discussion with your doctor at your next visit.

CHAPTER 2

What causes high cholesterol?

U nhealthy cholesterol levels don't just spring up overnight. Rather they happen by stealth over a much longer period of time. In some people however they may even be present from birth.

There are four main causes of high cholesterol:

Any one of these can be the single cause of your cholesterol levels being out of kilter, but together they can also act to unbalance your cholesterol levels even further.

- Increasing age
- Unhealthy diet and lifestyle
- The genes we inherit from our parents
- Other medical conditions or medicines you might be taking.

Age

Most people are not born with high cholesterol but it tends to increase as they get older. Very low levels of cholesterol are present in the cord blood of unborn babies, as low as 1.3–2.4 mmol/l. Once we are born and during early childhood, cholesterol levels increase rapidly until around six years of age, at which point the increase becomes more gradual. Cholesterol levels dip again during adolescence then progressively rise throughout adult life. In fact, studies have consistently shown that cholesterol levels continue to rise until the age of 65 in men and 75 in women. It is not fully understood why cholesterol increases with age but it is likely that the majority of the rise is related to diet, BMI (Body Mass Index) and other lifestyle changes such as decreasing activity and patterns of smoking.

There are also differences in the levels of cholesterol in men and women. On average, men aged 20–59 tend to have higher LDL-cholesterol levels when compared to women of the same age. However after the age of 30, and especially post-menopause, these differences in LDL cholesterol narrow so that, on average, by the age of 60 women tend to have higher LDL-cholesterol levels than men.

Boys and girls have similar HDL-cholesterol levels but after puberty these levels drop in men and remain lower than those in women. Men also tend to have smaller HDL particles compared to women.

Heart disease has long been considered a man's disease but women should never be complacent – far more women die of heart disease than breast cancer. It is a good idea to watch out for escalating cholesterol levels after the menopause, as there are often changes in the pattern of cholesterol around this time, which may be linked to the loss of the female hormone oestrogen.

Lifestyle

The way we live can also affect our cholesterol levels.

Diet

Diet can have a direct influence on cholesterol in several ways. We discuss diet in more detail later in this book in chapter 7. Chapters 6, 7 and 8 provide guidance and advice on reducing your own cholesterol by following our unique diet and lifestyle plan.

The typical British diet is far from healthy. Dietary surveys demonstrate that the average diet in the UK contains:

- Too much saturated fat
- Too few fruits and vegetables
- Too much salt
- Too many processed starchy and sugary foods
- Too few wholegrains.

Smoking

If you are a smoker you will already know that there are lots of good reasons for quitting. Smoking is well known to be an independent risk factor for heart disease. One of the effects of smoking is to reduce the levels of circulating HDL cholesterol (good cholesterol). This in turn reduces the protective effect that HDL cholesterol normally provides.

Smoking also produces numerous free radicals, which are harmful chemicals that result in circulating cholesterol becoming more atherogenic. Put simply the chemicals in cigarette smoke can damage the walls of blood vessels and result in harmful LDL-cholesterol particles accumulating in the walls of our arteries. This process is called **atherosclerosis** (see pages 37–42).

Being physically active

While smoking increases the risk of heart disease, being physically active has the opposite effect. By being more active you are able to:

- Burn up more dietary or stored fat
- Prevent excess calories being stored as fat
- Achieve and/or maintain a healthier weight
- Reduce and/or maintain a healthier waist circumference
- Increase your HDL cholesterol (good cholesterol) level

- Exercise your heart muscle
- Maintain a positive mood
- Reduce and manage stress levels
- Reduce risk of developing type 2 diabetes
- Improve blood sugar control in diabetics.

Alcohol

Alcohol has little direct effect on LDL cholesterol, but it does have some effects on HDL cholesterol and can increase blood triglyceride levels too. There is also little doubt that too much alcohol can do damage to your heart and circulatory system. Current guidelines call for restricting alcohol intake to no more than 3–4 standard units a day for men and 2–3 units a day for women. It is also important to have a couple of alcohol-free days each week and to avoid binge drinking.

Alcohol itself is high in calories. Gram for gram it contains almost twice as many calories as sugar.

Regular drinking above recommended amounts can:

- Increase your weight and waist circumference
- Increase your risk of high blood pressure, one of the most important risk factors for having a heart attack or a stroke
- Weaken the heart muscle, so the heart can't pump blood efficiently; eventually this can cause heart failure and result in premature death
- Increase the liver's output of triglycerides – another blood fat which is linked to cardiovascular disease
- Increase the levels of VLDL (see page 12) – a triglyceride and cholesterol-carrying particle that is linked to cardiovascular disease.

Alcohol in small amounts (around 1–2 units a day) can have a small positive effect on HDL-cholesterol levels. The effect is the same no matter what form the alcohol comes in. If you do drink already there is no reason to give it up completely unless your doctor has advised this. However if you don't drink, this positive effect is too small to justify starting to drink alcohol.

Genetic causes of high cholesterol

If genetic causes are fully or partly responsible for your high cholesterol then you may have been surprised to find out you have high cholesterol, especially if you consider yourself to have a healthy diet and lifestyle.

But high cholesterol and other lipid conditions can be inherited. So if one of your parents, a brother or a sister has high cholesterol this might be the reason you do too.

Researchers have identified more than 100 genes that can influence the levels of blood fats, including cholesterol, and the lipoproteins that carry them around our bodies. For many people, high cholesterol results from inheriting a specific genetic code from their parents, which influences cholesterol levels in the body. Yes it's true, you can have high cholesterol even if you have a very healthy diet, are a good weight, physically active and a non-smoker. Cholesterol can affect young people, men and women, people of all sizes and shapes, all ethnic groups and all nationalities. It simply does not discriminate. Sometimes just one 'altered' gene is enough to increase your cholesterol to dangerous levels. We estimate that between 1 in 200 to 1 in 500 people in the UK are affected by high cholesterol as a result of inheriting a single altered gene from their parent.

There are other ways you can inherit high cholesterol too. For example, the combined small effects of inheriting many genes that code for unhealthy high cholesterol levels is one of the most common causes of high cholesterol.

Familial hypercholesterolaemia (often shortened to FH)

Familial (family) **hyper** (high) **cholesterolaemia** (cholesterol in the blood) – is an inherited condition that leads to exceptionally high cholesterol levels, often double and sometimes four times that of the general population. Cholesterol levels are raised from birth, resulting in lifelong exposure to high cholesterol.

FH is not caused by an unhealthy lifestyle. It is passed from generation to generation through a 'faulty' or 'altered' gene. The pattern of inheritance is called 'autosomal dominant'. This means that an individual only needs one altered gene in order to have the condition. A child born to a mother or a father with FH has a one in two (50 per cent) chance of having the condition from the affected parent.

Left untreated, people with FH experience raised levels of cholesterol over many years and this can lead to early heart disease. Early diagnosis and effective treatment reduces the risk of heart disease and can help ensure that people with FH have a normal life expectancy.

About 1 in 500 people have FH, although some lipid experts believe it is more common than this, perhaps as high as 1 in 200. Very occasionally, someone is born with two altered genes because they inherit an altered gene from each parent. This happens in approximately one in a million births, affecting between 60–120 children and adults in the UK. Cholesterol levels are usually much higher in this form of FH and early diagnosis and treatment is vital. This form of FH is called homozygous FH or HoFH.

While a healthy diet and lifestyle are essential for people with FH, most also require treatment with a high-potency statin (or another potent cholesterol-lowering medical treatment) and regular follow-ups with a doctor who specialises in managing lipid conditions.

Familial combined hyperlipidaemia (FCH)

Often shortened to FCH, **familial** (family) combined **hyper** (high) **lipidaemia** (fats in the blood) is an inherited condition affecting around one person in every hundred.

Like FH, people with FCH are at increased risk of cardio-vascular disease and typically there is a history of premature heart disease or raised blood fats in close family members.

But unlike FH the pattern of raised fats is different. In FCH both triglycerides and cholesterol levels are raised. It is also unlikely that FCH is caused by a single gene alteration. More likely it is caused by a combination of genes working individu-ally, or together, to affect the levels of blood fats.

The levels of cholesterol and triglycerides can vary a lot and change over time in people with FCH and this often reflects changes in diet, lifestyle, body weight, alcohol intake and phys-ical activity.

As FCH is less well understood than FH it is not so easy to diagnose. Triglycerides and cholesterol may not be raised until the age of 20 or 30.

People with FCH have a unique pattern of raised fats:

- Raised levels of VLDL particles (these are triglyceride-rich particles produced by the liver)
- Elevated ApoB levels (each VLDL particle contains one particle of ApoB, so more VLDL means more ApoB)
- Raised fasting triglyceride levels
- LDL-cholesterol particles that are smaller and more compact (dense) than normal.

People with FH and FCH should, ideally, be diagnosed and treated in a lipid clinic with access to regular follow-ups.

Screening family members

Because of the increased risk of cardiovascular disease, all first-degree relatives (brothers, sisters, children) of people with FH or FCH should be screened to check if they have inherited the same genetic condition. In most cases a lipid clinic is the best place to do this. It is possible to diagnose FH with a genetic test but at the time of writing this is not available in all areas of the UK.

Polygenic

Polygenic literally means 'many genes'. This is the most commonly inherited cause of raised cholesterol in the UK and is caused by the small effects of many genes combining to raise overall cholesterol levels. Traditionally, high cholesterol has been defined as a total cholesterol level over 5 mmol/l. On this basis around 50 per cent of middle-aged men and women have raised cholesterol which is polygenic in origin.

There is much debate about when doctors should intervene with statins for people with polygenic high cholesterol. Most have agreed that the deciding factor is overall cardiovascular risk (the sum of all a person's risk factors). It is easy to determine overall cardiovascular risk (see the section starting on page 43 for details).

Secondary causes of altered blood fats

An underactive thyroid gland

Often called hypothyroidism, this condition affects around 2 per cent of women and usually increases with age, reaching a peak at about 60 years old. It is rather less prevalent in men. A milder form of hypothyroidism, sometimes called subclinical hypothyroidism, affects up to four times as many women (8 per cent) and up to 3 per cent of men.

Both forms of hypothyroidism tend to result in increased levels of total cholesterol, LDL cholesterol and sometimes triglycerides too, although levels are usually lower with the subclinical form. HDL-cholesterol levels may also be raised. These effects are often reversed with appropriate thyroxin replacement therapy.

A blood test is usually conducted by your doctor to check for levels of TSH (thyroid stimulating hormone) and free thyroxin to determine a diagnosis of hypothyroidism as the root cause of raised blood fats.

Kidney diseases

Raised cholesterol and triglycerides often occur in people with varying degrees of kidney disease.

Nephrotic syndrome

This occurs when the filters in the kidneys, which are responsible for filtering waste products from the bloodstream, become 'leaky'. This means that proteins are able to leak out into the urine, whereas normally urine contains virtually no protein. Nephrotic syndrome has a number of causes, some of which are more successfully treated than others. The main symptom is fluid retention but people usually have raised levels of cholesterol and other blood fats too.

Kidney Failure

Blood fats, including cholesterol and triglycerides, are often altered in people at all stages of kidney failure and can be made worse by dialysis treatment. As cardiovascular disease is common in people with kidney failure, statins and other cholesterol-lowering medications are often prescribed. Blood fats often return closer to normal levels after transplantation, especially if good kidney function is achieved.

Liver

The liver is the powerhouse for lipid metabolism and so any conditions that affect the liver can also cause raised cholesterol and triglycerides. Bile, a secretion produced from cholesterol breakdown in the liver, is stored in the gall bladder and expelled through the bile duct into the gut in response to mealtimes. Any blockage in the production of bile or its mechanical release into the gut can cause raised blood cholesterol, for example, blocking of the bile duct caused by cholesterol stones or other organs pressing on the bile duct. There is little or no evidence that the development of gallstones (which are formed from crystallised cholesterol) is associated with coronary heart disease.

Obesity

Abdominal obesity is strongly associated with an unhealthy pattern of blood fats, such as raised LDL cholesterol, low levels of the protective HDL cholesterol and raised triglycerides. These changes result from insulin resistance. It is estimated that around a third of people with a BMI over 27 have high cholesterol. While weight gain increases cholesterol levels, weight loss can bring about moderate reductions in cholesterol and other blood fats. On average, a 10 per cent weight loss can lower LDL cholesterol by about 15 per cent, total cholesterol by 10 per cent and increase HDL cholesterol by 8 per cent.

While weight loss is recommended, it is vitally important that new healthy habits are also formed to help ensure that any weight loss is maintained.

Diabetes

Impaired sugar tolerance and type 2 diabetes are often the consequences of obesity especially in those who are genetically more predisposed to developing diabetes. Approximately 85 per cent of type 2 diabetics are obese or overweight. Insulin resistance is the main defect in diabetes and metabolic syndrome (a combination of physical and biochemical characteristics putting a person at higher risk of diabetes and cardiovascular disease – it includes high blood pressure, abdominal obesity, and raised blood fats). People with type 2 diabetes often show a typical pattern of slightly raised or normal LDL cholesterol levels, raised triglycerides and low-HDL cholesterol. Although LDL levels may not be raised very much in diabetics the LDL taxis themselves are often abnormal (smaller and denser) which makes them more likely to cause problems.

Medications

Several commonly prescribed medicines also affect blood cholesterol and triglyceride levels. The main effects are described below.

Drug	Triglycerides	LDL Cholesterol	HDL Cholesterol
Thiazide Diuretics	Increase	Increase	No effect
B Blockers	Some increase		Some decrease
Oestrogens	Increase		Increase
Androgens (steroids)	Decrease	Increase	Decrease
Progestogens		Increase	Decrease
HIV retroviral therapy	Increase	Increase	

Signs and symptoms

It is almost impossible to know you have high cholesterol without having a blood test as there are very few signs and symptoms.

Many years of exposure to high cholesterol can result in some subtle outward signs, but these are often difficult to find. Even doctors, unless they know what they are looking for, might overlook them. These outward signs, when they occur, result from cholesterol being deposited in soft tissues in the hands, feet and in and around the eyes.

Outward signs to look for:

Where on the body	Medical name	Description
Eyes	Corneal arcus	A white ring around the iris, the coloured part of the eye
Eyes	Xanthelasma	One or more flat growths outside the eyelid, often yellowish in colour and composed of fatty material
Hands and ankles	Tendon Xanthomas	Cholesterol deposits in the tendons, which show as whitish/yellowish swellings on the knuckles, or the Achilles tendon at the back of the ankle

Most people won't notice or experience any symptoms – all the more reason to ask your doctor for a routine blood test to determine your cholesterol levels. This is especially important if you have reason to believe you may have high cholesterol. For example, do you have close family members with high cholesterol or have any of your close family had symptoms of cardiovascular disease – heart attack, angina, stroke – at an early age (before 60 years in a woman or 50 years in a man)? Even if your cholesterol test results were normal the last time they were measured, it's a good idea to repeat the process every five years.

In this chapter we have concentrated on the causes of high cholesterol which are many and varied. A very large proportion of the adult UK population have cholesterol levels above the generally accepted healthy target of 5 mmol/l. In the next chapter we discuss why this matters and how cardiovascular disease develops.

CHAPTER 3

What is cardiovascular disease?

Today cardiovascular disease (CVD) is one of the UK and Ireland's biggest killers, accounting for a third of all deaths. Cardiovascular disease includes stroke, coronary heart disease (CHD) and other diseases of the circulatory system, such as peripheral arterial disease (PAD), which affects the legs and causes pain on walking, and some forms of kidney disease. CHD is by far the main contributor to CVD. On its own it accounts for over 14 per cent of all deaths compared to the next biggest killers of respiratory disease (13 per cent), stroke (9 per cent) and lung cancer (6 per cent). In comparison, breast cancer is responsible for 2 per cent of all deaths each year.

More tragic is the fact that cardiovascular diseases are the most common cause of premature death (before the age of 75), accounting for 28 per cent of all premature deaths in men and 19 per cent in women. CHD alone is responsible for 17 per cent of premature deaths in men and 8 per cent in women.

What exactly causes cardiovascular disease?

CVD is a chronic disease. It does not happen overnight. It is the result of a gradual process called atherosclerosis.

Atherosclerosis is a progressive condition which starts when we are young and continues throughout our lives. It affects absolutely everyone but to varying degrees. The speed at which it progresses is influenced by the number of risk factors an individual has. It is a complicated inflammatory disease that can be broken into three main stages:

Stage 1: Damage to blood vessel wall

The first stage is when damage occurs to the inside of the lining of the blood vessel wall. The cause of this initial damage can result from mechanical, biochemical or toxic effects (such as high blood pressure, environmental pollutants or smoking). This initial damage causes an inflammatory reaction (similar to if you grazed your knee) with white blood cells being attracted to the area of damage. White blood cells are part of the body's normal protective systems.

These white blood cells enter the lining of the blood vessel wall where the damage has taken place, also allowing the entry of cholesterol-laden LDL particles. In their attempt to help heal the damage, the white blood cells feast on the LDL particles, and become engorged with fat. At the same time, smooth muscle cells migrate into the space to help heal the damage. This produces a fibrous matrix of proteins that make a protective, fibre-filled cap over the damage (just like a scab on your knee). It is the combination of this matrix of proteins and the accumulation of fat-filled cells that make up a fatty streak. Fatty streaks are the first signs of atherosclerosis.

While atherosclerosis can occur in any blood vessel in the body, it is of most concern in smaller blood vessels that provide a critical supply of blood to the body's major organs, such as the heart and lungs, and parts of the body such as the brain and legs. It is not possible to detect fatty steaks through routine testing but they have been found in young people who have died prematurely from other causes.

Stage 2: The inside of the blood vessel starts to narrow

Just like a graze to your knee, many of these areas of damage heal naturally. Sometimes, however, the tissue can become thickened and a fatty plaque develops. As a result the artery can start to change shape.

Over time, the plaque expands and starts to protrude into the inner artery space causing the blood vessel to narrow.

In addition, plaque hardens over time, causing the arterial walls to thicken and harden, severely reducing their elasticity and fluidity. This lack of elasticity in the artery can also cause raised blood pressure, another risk factor for heart disease.

Stage 3: Arteries become severely narrowed

Eventually the inner lining of the blood vessel may burst. This triggers the clotting process inside the blood vessel known as thrombosis. The damaged area or clot usually heals over time and becomes incorporated into the plaque. However sometimes a clot can break free and begin to travel around the body. This is called an embolus and can be very dangerous.

Over many years there can be *excessive* narrowing of the arteries, meaning that less blood can flow through them. This excessive narrowing can be detected on some forms of X-ray but these tests are not usually carried out unless symptoms alert your doctor to the presence of narrowed arteries.

The symptoms of atherosclerosis become more common as we get older. But most people don't know this slow process of atherosclerosis is going on inside them until they develop severe symptoms such as angina or intermittent claudication (pain on walking), or even have a stroke or heart attack.

The symptoms a person experiences are determined by where the atherosclerosis occurs in the body and the extent of the blockage. For example, a narrowing of any of the three small coronary arteries that feed the heart muscle can lead to angina or to a heart attack if the artery is completely blocked. A blockage in an artery leading to the brain would cause a stroke and a blockage in an artery that feeds muscles in the legs can cause pain when walking.

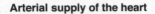

Arterial supply of the heart

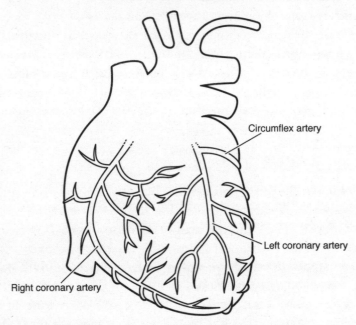

Illustration of a heart with 3 coronary arteries

Angina is an uncomfortable feeling, tightness or pain in the chest which usually occurs during exercise or when stressed. The pain may spread to the arms, neck, jaw, back or stomach. It occurs because one or more of the coronary arteries in the heart are narrowed, restricting the flow of blood to the heart muscle. You might experience angina if it is a cold day or if you are walking after a meal. The symptoms are not the same for everyone and for some it may be confused with heartburn.

An angina attack can vary in length from 30 seconds to several minutes, but most attacks last only a few minutes. Your doctor will most likely prescribe a medicine that improves your symptoms rapidly, usually within five minutes. The most common of these is a glyceryl trinitrate spray. Angina that occurs more frequently and is triggered by ever decreasing levels of physical activity is known as unstable angina. It may occur at minimal activity, at rest, or even wake you up when sleeping. Symptoms of angina can be controlled with the appropriate medication. If the pain persists, despite taking glyceryl trinitrate over 15 minutes, then you should call 999.

Heart attack or myocardial infarction (MI) occurs when the blood supply to a part of the heart is completely blocked, causing part of the heart to be damaged or to die. Symptoms can include chest pain or pain in other parts of the body, such as pain travelling from the chest to the arms, jaw, neck, back and abdomen. It can include symptoms of dizziness or feeling light-headed, sweating or shortness of breath. Although the chest pain is often severe, some people may only experience minor pain. You should dial 999 immediately if you suspect that you or someone you know is having a heart attack.

Stroke occurs when the blood supply to part of the brain is cut off, for example, if a blood clot blocks an artery that carries blood to your brain. Without a blood supply, the brain cells can be damaged or destroyed, so a stroke can affect the way your body or mind will function in the future. The signs and symptoms of a stroke vary from person to person but usually begin suddenly. The main stroke symptoms can be remembered using the well know acronym FAST which stands for Face-Arms-Speech-Time.

- Face: has the face dropped on one side?
- Arms: can the person with suspected stroke lift both arms above their head?
- Speech: is their speech slurred?
- Time: act now – it is time to dial 999 immediately if you see any of these signs or symptoms. Any delay can have serious consequences and may be fatal.

Peripheral Arterial disease (PAD) is usually associated with a narrowing of the arteries in the legs. It can cause calf pain especially when walking. PAD may also affect other arteries such as the abdominal aorta, the carotid arteries (in the neck) or the iliac arteries (near your pelvis).

**Excess cholesterol
accumulating in arteries**

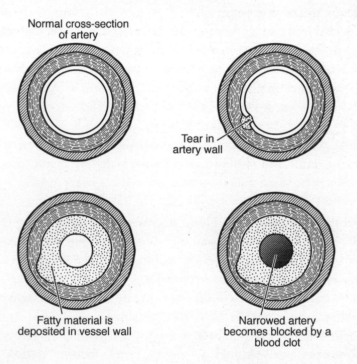

Normal cross-section
of artery

Tear in
artery wall

Fatty material is
deposited in vessel wall

Narrowed artery
becomes blocked by a
blood clot

Before we move on to the next section, be sure that you have grasped the main concepts above. It's important to understand that cardiovascular disease is a slow progressive disorder and that it is caused by a process called atherosclerosis. In the next section we start to understand the main factors that drive this process of atherosclerosis.

Who is at risk?

Having unhealthy levels of cholesterol (such as high cholesterol, or a combination of low HDL cholesterol with raised triglycerides) is only one risk factor for cardiovascular disease (CVD).

There are many other factors that influence your risk of developing CVD, and it is the sum of these that determines your overall risk. The more risk factors you have the more likely you are to develop CVD.

Many doctors communicate cardiovascular risk by referring to the risk of having a heart attack or stroke over a 10-year period. This is usually expressed as a percentage. A 20 per cent risk means a one in five chance of having a stroke or heart attack in the next 10 years and is considered high risk. Moderate risk is 10–20 per cent and low risk less than 10 per cent. Doctors encourage people at high or moderate risk to take a statin and to make any necessary lifestyle changes to bring their overall risk down.

While this approach has a lot of merit it does not take account of the fact that most heart attacks are 30–40 years in the making. For example, a person aged 35 who is a smoker and has high LDL cholesterol but no other risk factors, might be at low risk of having a heart attack or stroke in the next 10 years, so they have a low 'absolute risk'. However, when compared to someone of the same age and same risk profile but who is a non-smoker and has low LDL-cholesterol levels, the first person is at high 'relative risk'. In other words, their chances of experiencing premature heart disease in the long term, and before the age of 65, are high.

Doctors are increasingly looking for those people who are at high lifetime risk of CVD so that they can be helped at an early age before they develop active disease. New risk calculators are now available which can help identify people at high lifetime risk as well as high 10-year risk. Not only this, they can also estimate how many years a heart attack or stroke might be delayed by an intervention such as stopping smoking, taking a statin, or managing high blood pressure.

Where can I calculate my own risk?

The Joint British Societies have developed a risk calculator for health professionals that can be used by individuals too. It has been designed to indicate your lifelong risk of heart disease or stroke and when your first heart attack or stroke might happen if you do nothing. You can access this online by using the search term JBS3, and there is also a handy app to use on your iPhone. Another way to do this is by using the online heart age tool. This will also tell you how 'old' your heart is compared to your own age. You can access this at www.heartage.co.uk or www.heartage.me

What are the main risk factors for cardiovascular disease?

It is helpful to divide the main risk factors into two groups: non-modifiable (things you cannot influence) and modifiable (things that you can influence).

Risk factors for coronary heart disease (CHD)

Non-modifiable risk factors (can't be changed)	Modifiable risk factors (can be changed)
Existing CHD	High blood pressure
Family history of heart disease	Raised or unhealthy blood fats (cholesterol, triglycerides)
Age	Diabetes
Being male	Being overweight or obese
Ethnic factors	Smoking
	Being inactive
	Excessive alcohol
	Stress

WHAT IS CARDIOVASCULAR DISEASE?

Non-modifiable risk factors

Existing CHD

This should be fairly self-explanatory but just to reiterate: if you have already developed heart disease, for example, if you have had a heart attack, have angina or been diagnosed with coronary heart disease, then you are at high risk of having a heart attack or stroke in the future. If this is the situation then it is very important to manage all other risk factors and in the process help prevent any further coronary events. Most people at high risk will be prescribed a cholesterol-lowering drug, such as a statin, and it's important that you take it. We talk more about statins in chapter 9. At the same time you can help improve your health by following the other lifestyle steps outlined in this book.

Age

As we get older our risk of cardiovascular disease gradually increases. Age is by far the biggest determinant of cardiovascular disease.

Gender

Before the age of 60, men are at greater risk than women. This is because before the menopause women receive some protection from the female hormone oestrogen. On average women go through the menopause around the age of 50. Once past the menopause, the gap between men and women quickly narrows.

Ethnic origin

Some ethnic groups are at increased cardiovascular risk than others. For example, people who are directly descended from South Asia (India, Bangladesh, Pakistan) are at increased risk of heart disease and diabetes. Similarly direct descendants of

Afro-Caribbean populations are at increased risk of high blood pressure and stroke when compared to the average Caucasian person living in Britain.

Family history

Early heart or circulatory disease in close (first-degree) family members. This includes parents, grandparents, brothers and sisters, and can indicate an inherited vulnerability to cardio-vascular disease. So it's a good idea to find out, if you can, if other family members have heart or circulatory disease or high cholesterol and if so at what age they developed this. It's impor-tant to share this with your doctor, especially if it occurred before the age of 55 in a male relative or 65 in a female rela-tive. Early disease might be explained by other risk factors such as smoking or diabetes, so find out about these too.

Modifiable risk factors

High blood pressure (hypertension)

Blood pressure is a measure of the force of blood as it is pumped around the body. It is recorded as two numbers: the systolic records the pressure when the heart beats and the dias-tolic when the heart is at rest between beats. Both numbers are important. It is measured in millimetres of mercury, which is written down as mmHg.

Normal blood pressure is considered to be:

- Systolic – between 110 and 130
- Diastolic – between 85 and 60.

High blood pressure, or hypertension, is diagnosed when several readings show your

- Systolic pressure is 140 or above
- Your diastolic is 90 or above
- Or both.

High blood pressure tends to run in families, but blood pressure is also influenced by lifestyle; it may even be raised as a result of a visit to the doctor if you are anxious.

To prevent blood pressure from rising, it is important to achieve and maintain a healthy body weight, keep alcohol intake moderate, reduce salt intake, manage and reduce stress levels and be physically active.

Why is high blood pressure (hypertension) dangerous?

High blood pressure can put a strain on your heart, blood vessels and kidneys. If your blood pressure remains high for a long time it can damage your arteries, put extra strain on the heart muscle and increase the risk of heart attacks and stroke. High blood pressure contributes to more than a fifth of heart attacks and half of all strokes. Lowering your blood pressure reduces these risks. If your blood pressure is too high your GP will prescribe medication and review this regularly. However, simple changes to your diet and lifestyle can also be a very effective part of treatment.

Unhealthy Patterns of Blood fats

Cholesterol

As discussed in chapter 1 there are many medical conditions and treatments that give rise to one, or a combination of, the following: raised LDL cholesterol, lowered HDL cholesterol and small dense LDL particles.

Doctors now refer to these altered patterns of blood fats as dyslipidaemia. Having one or more of the above can be harmful because they are associated with an increased chance of developing some types of cardiovascular disease, such as heart disease, stroke and peripheral arterial disease.

Triglycerides

High blood triglycerides are also associated with an increased risk of developing coronary heart disease. A low level of HDL cholesterol and more dense particles of LDL cholesterol usually accompany raised triglycerides, and this pattern of blood lipids is often seen in people with diabetes or pre-diabetes. This pattern of blood lipids is believed to be more toxic to the linings of our arteries.

Raised triglycerides, often referred to as hypertriglyceridaemia, are often accompanied by changes in blood-clotting mechanisms.

Individuals can be born with genetic defects of triglyceride metabolism. Although rare this can result in very high fasting triglyceride levels, usually above 10 mmol/l. When triglyceride levels are so high the main danger can be pancreatitis (inflammation of the pancreas gland) and not necessarily an increased susceptibility to heart disease.

Triglycerides can also be raised because of excessive alcohol intake.

Diabetes

Diabetes is a condition where the body is either resistant to the effects of insulin or does not produce enough of it. Insulin, a hormone produced by the pancreas, is necessary to unlock the body's cells, letting sugar in so that it can be used for energy. Because sugar cannot get into the cell it builds up in the blood stream above normal levels.

Over time too much sugar in the blood damages the arteries, causing them to become stiff and hard. The amount of fat in the blood also increases in diabetes. Large amounts of fat are released from the body's fat stores to provide energy to compensate. Uncontrolled diabetes also results in low levels of lipoprotein lipase, an enzyme that normally helps to clear fat from the blood after a meal.

This pattern of high blood sugars and fats puts people with diabetes at elevated risk of heart disease.

Smoking

Tobacco, regardless of whether it is smoked or chewed, causes a number of problems that increase overall cardiovascular risk. In particular it:

- Speeds up the process of atherosclerosis, which as we have seen on pages 37–42, is a process that damages the walls of blood vessels, causing inflammation and resulting in cholesterol becoming trapped in the artery wall. This eventually causes the blood vessel to become narrowed
- Temporarily raises blood pressure
- Lowers the capacity for exercise due to a decrease in the amount of oxygen that the blood can carry
- Increases the tendency for blood to clot which may result in a heart attack or a stroke if clots prevent blood circulating to a part of the brain or the heart.

Even after having smoked for many years, stopping smoking will reduce CHD risk. After five years, your risk of having a heart attack falls to about half that of a smoker. Research also shows that non-smokers who live with smokers have a greater risk of CHD than other non-smokers.

How harmful is shisha smoking?

Tobacco smoking in whatever form is harmful. Shisha smoking, also called hookah or hubble-bubble smoking, is an unusual way of smoking tobacco, sometimes mixed with fruit or sugar molasses through a bowl and hose or a tube. Although traditionally smoked in the Middle East, it is becoming increasingly popular in the UK. People who smoke shisha tend to do so for much longer periods of time than they smoke a cigarette. One puff of shisha delivers the same amount of smoke as you would get from smoking a whole cigarette!

Being inactive

Increasing your activity is one way of cutting your risk of CHD. Cardiovascular benefits of regular physical activity include reduced blood pressure, improved weight control, improved cholesterol levels, reduced risk of diabetes and, if diabetic, better blood sugar control. Exercise is also a good way of relieving stress and exercising the heart muscle.

For health benefits, you should be aiming for at least 150 minutes of moderate-intensity physical activity per week. Walking, swimming, cycling, jogging and dancing are all excellent choices. Try to spread the 150 minutes across the week, for example five sessions of 30 minutes.

Excessive alcohol

Alcohol in moderation may very slightly reduce the risk of heart disease in men over 40 years old and in women who have gone through menopause. However, excessive consumption can directly damage the heart muscle and can cause irregular beating of the heart. Alcohol can also contribute to weight gain, high triglycerides, high blood pressure, stroke and cancer.

Men should drink no more than 28 units per week and women no more than 21 units per week (see pages 104–5).

Stress

We all feel stress but it affects us in different ways and we each respond differently. Some individuals may not even realise how much stress they are under.

For most people, a certain amount of stress is healthy in that it can help keep them alert and motivated. However, as stress levels build, especially if they remain high for long periods, they can be harmful to health.

Examples of common responses to stress include disturbed sleep patterns, headaches, chest discomfort, irritability and restlessness. People who are more stressed may use coping mechanisms such as smoking, over-eating, under-eating or poor eating, excessive drinking or taking prescribed medicines such as antidepressants.

Stress can also exacerbate symptoms in people with pre-existing heart disease, and what's more it can contribute to high blood pressure. In addition, the amount of stress you have, and how you deal with it, can influence your risk of developing CVD. See chapter 8 on managing your stress levels.

By now you should have a better understanding of CVD and what causes it as well as the main modifiable risk factors. In the next few chapters we will start to address some practical ways to help you identify how you could start to make some small changes to how you live your life, with the aim of reducing your overall cardiovascular risk.

CHAPTER 4

Managing your weight

Weight gain, leading to obesity, is a huge health issue and obesity is now recognised as the biggest cause of ill health in the UK today. Obesity has far-reaching consequences for everyone, not just the individual people it affects and their families. There are wide-ranging implications for an overstretched NHS, industry, employers and the British economy. It's a major health and economic challenge!

The average Briton today is much heavier than the generation before them; in fact, it is fast becoming normal to be overweight and Britain is becoming an obese society. Added to that, our perceptions of what being overweight looks like have changed too.

It's not that people have less willpower or that our biology has changed; it's the environment we find ourselves in that has changed. Scientists now describe the Western world as an 'obesogenic environment'. This means that there are many factors that conspire together to encourage weight gain. Our work patterns, the way we get about, our leisure pursuits, abundant food choice and food availability have all seen radical change over the last three generations. When coupled with the underlying tendency that many of us have to gain weight and retain it, the result is hardly surprising.

Not only are the causes of obesity complex, but the problem is also very difficult to solve. The rise in obesity is worldwide and no country has yet developed a comprehensive long-term strategy to tackle it. While governments are responsible for the overall health and well-being of their populations, individuals have a personal responsibility for their own health and there is much we all can do to reach, and then maintain, a healthier weight. The good news is that obesity doesn't need to be inevitable.

Why worry about your weight?

We all like to look and feel good. Being a healthy weight and shape are an integral part of feeling great and the confidence it brings. But could your weight be affecting your health too?

Careful observation of populations around the world tells us that being obese reduces the number of years we can expect to live. Conversely losing weight, and maintaining that weight loss, can increase our life expectancy.

Excess weight is one of the top risk factors for ill health and is linked to the risk of type 2 diabetes, high blood pressure, stroke and coronary heart disease, as well as some types of cancer. It can also aggravate existing back and joint pain, limit mobility and increase breathlessness. Of particular concern is fat stored around the waist, which is metabolically more active than fat stored in other parts of the body.

Am I obese or overweight?

Being obese or overweight is usually defined by reference to the Body Mass Index (BMI). You can calculate your own BMI very easily. To do this you will need your weight in kilogrammes and your height in metres. Simply divide your weight in kilograms by your height in metres squared (metres × metres). For example, a man with a height of 1.6 metres and a weight of 90 kilogrammes would have a BMI of 35.1

BMI = weight in kilogrammes ÷ [height in metres ×
                                    height in metres]

BMI = 90 ÷ [1.6 × 1.6]

BMI = 90 ÷ 2.56

BMI = 35.1

Overweight is usually defined as a BMI of 25–29.9 but health professionals increasingly recognise that for people of South Asian origin a BMI above 23 should be defined as overweight, as it is associated with higher risk in that population.

Obesity is defined as a BMI above 30.

But BMI is not a foolproof measure of body composition. It falls down in some cases, for example, it cannot accurately assess body fat in those individuals with higher than average muscle mass such as sportsmen and women.

Waist circumference and cardiovascular disease risk

Where excess fat is stored on the body is also key to the development of insulin resistance and cardiovascular disease (CVD). Usually we store fat in our adipose tissues, which are located below the skin and around our major organs. Under normal circumstances the inside of our organs contain little or no fat.

However, in some situations (usually driven by our genetics and our lifestyle), fat can become trapped inside our organs, for example, the liver or pancreas. Here it can interfere with how these organs function, disrupting the normal metabolic processes. Fat present in the liver and other major organs is usually referred to as ectopic fat. It is not easy to determine how much ectopic fat a person has by looking at them. However, a person's waist circumference provides a good measure of abdominal fat. Abdominal fat includes fat stored under skin (subcutaneous fat), fat stored around our organs (visceral fat) and fat stored within the liver and pancreas (ectopic fat). So a greater waist circumference is an indicator of a greater amount of disruptive ectopic fat. However, it is very possible that two people with the same waist measurement may have widely differing proportions of subcutaneous, visceral and ectopic fat to each other. Despite this, it is widely accepted by health professionals that abdominal fat is an indicator of increased risk when compared to fat stored around the hips or lower body.

The best way to measure abdominal fat is by measuring waist circumference. The waist should be measured at roughly the widest point. Scientists agree that a waist measurement over 88 cm in a woman and 102 cm in a man is an indicator of increased risk.

The good news is that when people do lose weight, much of the initial weight loss appears to come from abdominal fat. An overweight individual who is able to lose just 5 per cent of their body fat could lose around 30–40 per cent of their abdominal fat.

What would achieving a 5 or 10 per cent weight loss look like?

Weight in stones	5 per cent weight loss	10 per cent weight loss	Weight in KG	5 per cent weight loss	10 per cent weight loss
12	8.5 lbs	1stone 3 lbs	75	3.75 kg	7.5 kg
13	9 lbs	1 stone 4 lbs	80	4 kg	8 kg
14	10 lbs	1 stone 6 lbs	85	4.25 kg	8.5 kg
15	10.5 lbs	1 stone 7 lbs	90	4.5 kg	9 kg
16	11 lbs	1 stone 8 lbs	95	4.75 kg	9.5 kg
17	12 lbs	1 stone 10 lbs	100	5 kg	10 kg
18	13 lbs	1stone 11 lbs	105	5.25 kg	10.5 kg
19	13 lbs	1 stone 13 lbs	110	5.5 kg	11 kg
20	1 stone	2 stones	115	5.75 kg	11.5 kg

Even on its own, physical activity may be able to reduce waist circumference and abdominal fat. A study published in the *Journal of the American Medical Association* in 2003 showed that moderate activity of just 30 minutes a day could prevent weight gain, promote modest weight loss, loss of abdominal fat and improve fitness. They showed that the greater the activity, the greater the weight loss and reduction in waist circumference.

Exercise without weight loss is also far from failure. Why? Because regular physical activity can reduce waist circumference and alter fat distribution around the body even if weight is unaffected. In a 2008 publication of a well-known Canadian journal, researchers reviewed the effects of many exercise interventions on the health of overweight individuals and concluded that changes in body composition, and not body weight, were most meaningful in bringing about improvements in insulin sensitivity. They argued that **decreases** in body fat often occur at the same time as similar **increases** in muscle tissue when people increase their physical activity. These similar, but opposite, effects often cancel each other out when you put someone on the scales. Their results indicated that, although many studies show little change in overall weight, significant decreases in waist circumference and improvements in cardiovascular risk factors resulted from increasing physical activity.

In the UK we are encouraged to do a minimum of 150 minutes of moderate activity every week. This works out at an average of 30 minutes over five days of the week. In order to reduce waist circumference, however, we need to work harder. The consensus is that at least 50–60 minutes per day is necessary.

You can easily measure your own waist circumference. Using a flexible tape measure or a piece of string, measure your waist at the midpoint between your lower ribs and the top of your pelvis. On most people this is around the umbilicus or tummy button, which in some people may not be the narrowest part of your waist. When you have your result, compare it against the recommendations in the following table.

Increased health risks associated with waist circumference

	Men	South-Asian men	Women
Increased health risk	Above 94 cm (37 in)	Above 90 cm (36 in)	Above 82 cm (32 in)
Serious health risk	Above 102 cm (40 in)	Above 90 cm (36 in)	Above 88 cm (35 in)

The benefits from losing just 5–10 per cent of your weight:

- Reduced blood pressure
- Improved blood glucose levels
- Reduced blood triglyceride levels
- Reduced LDL (bad cholesterol) levels
- Raised HDL (good cholesterol) levels
- Easier to move around
- Improved self-confidence and self-esteem.

Weight loss

Weight-loss advice is built upon the understanding that weight loss only occurs when you use up more energy (measured in kilocalories or kilojoules) than your body takes in from food and drink.

Losing weight steadily and gradually is safer, and the weight is much more likely to stay off, than if you lose it quickly. Aim for a weight loss of no more than 0.5–1 kg (1–2 pounds) a week. Eating a healthy diet with fewer calories, combined with more physical activity, achieves the best results.

Energy savings usually come from smaller portions and eating a diet that is lower in fat, alcohol and simple carbohydrates such as sugars. As fat and alcohol are high in calories it is especially important to limit these. There is also an emphasis on removing foods from the diet that contribute energy but provide few vitamins and minerals. This includes sugary drinks, confectionery as well as cakes, biscuits and puddings.

Energy provided by each of the four major food categories

- 1 gram of fat = 9 calories
- 1 gram of carbohydrate = 4 calories
- 1 gram of protein = 4 calories
- 1 gram of alcohol = 7 calories

The diet we recommend for weight loss is no different from the one we recommend for heart health. The only difference comes in ensuring a deficit in calories. Ideally you want to aim for a 500-kilocalorie difference between your daily calorie requirement (how many calories you use) and your daily calorie intake (how many calories you get from food or drink). That's where the joint approach of reducing energy intake from food and increasing physical activity at the same time comes in. About half of the calorie deficit comes from reducing food energy and half from increasing physical activity.

What works well for successful weight loss

People who lose weight successfully	People who don't lose weight or don't maintain their weight loss
Adopt a positive 'can do' attitude to weight loss	Adopt a negative 'can't do' attitude to weight loss
Set realistic expectations for weight loss over a prolonged period of time	Expect a quick fix and rapid weight loss and often adopt fad diets or extreme approaches
Understand, realise and value the true benefits for themselves of losing weight and engage with the process	Are not engaged with losing weight and are perhaps responding to the concerns of other family members or health professionals
Become more active, eat more healthily, choose smaller portions	Don't increase their levels of physical activity or don't maintain new activities
Eat regularly and have few snacks	Miss meals, including breakfast, and as a result snack more often
Make small changes to their own dietary patterns and establish new healthier habits gradually	Attempt a rigid dietary pattern which does not reflect normal eating or fit with their normal lifestyle

People who lose weight successfully	People who don't lose weight or don't maintain their weight loss
Change the way food is prepared and limit takeaways, eating out, and manage other eating occasions	Are often conflicted by eating occasions (meals out, family meals, food given as present) and do not plan how to manage these situations
Adopt a positive approach to relapses by learning new strategies	See relapses as negative and as a result often slip back into old habits
Identify triggers to problem eating and work to avoid or overcome them	Eat inappropriately in response to emotions or dietary triggers without confronting the causes
Share plans with friends and family and actively seek their support	Don't share their plans to lose weight with close friends and family and don't enlist their support
Are more flexible and relaxed in their dietary patterns and preferences. Food becomes less important in their lives. They allow themselves small amounts of their favourite foods from time to time.	Feel deprived, a victim of their weight and are resentful that they cannot eat what they want to
Learn new skills to enable them to plan, prepare and cook healthier meals	Are reluctant to develop new skills to plan, prepare and cook healthier meals

Options for weight loss

As mentioned above, the good news is that losing just 5 to 10 per cent of your weight can make a significant difference to your health. For most people, a 5–10 per cent weight loss is very achievable, realistic and should be possible to maintain over the long term. There are lots of approaches to weight loss and we cannot describe all of them here. As for any lifestyle change the process is the same, so you might like to look at chapter 6 on motivation to help you along the way.

There are many different ways of losing weight – some more healthy and efficacious than others. Remember that there are no quick fixes, and to lose weight healthily, you need to lose no more than 0.5–1 kg (1–2 pounds) a week.

Increasing activity

Increasing the amount of physical activity you do is an important part of weight loss and weight maintenance, as it increases your overall energy expenditure. This increase results from the effort of the physical activity itself, but also as a result of an increase in overall muscle mass. Muscle mass influences and contributes to the rate at which your body burns up energy. See chapter 8 on exercise.

Calorie restriction and portion control

Overall calorie restriction below that needed for everyday activities will, over time, result in weight loss. To achieve a ½-1 kilogramme (1–2 pound) loss over a week, a deficit of around 500–600 calories per day is needed. This deficit in calories (the difference between energy intake and energy expenditure) can come partly from reduced food consumption (reducing portion sizes, modifying intake of high fat and sugar containing foods) and partly from an increase in physical activity. To help identify changes you can make to your own diet, keep a food and activity diary over a typical week and then assess what changes can realistically be made.

Seek professional advice

Visit your GP to find out how they can support your weight loss. In some instances your doctor may be able to refer you to a registered dietitian for more tailored advice and support.

Your GP may have access to 'slimming or exercise on referral schemes' or in-house weight-loss programmes. In some cases your GP may be willing to prescribe Xenical (Orlistat). This is a medicine that helps support your weight loss. It works by preventing the absorption of about one third of the fat eaten at a meal. This means that fat passes through your body undigested. However, it only works safely and effectively if it is taken as part of a healthy energy-restricted, low-fat eating plan. Failing to restrict fat intake can result in unpleasant side effects such as flatulence, liquid oily stools and the need to find a toilet urgently.

Not everyone can take Xenical however. It is usually only available on prescription for people with serious weight problems; your doctor will advise if it is suitable for you.

Quick-Fix Diets

Magazines, books, newspapers and websites are constantly promoting the latest dietary fad. We don't recommend these. Sadly there is no magic formula for weight loss – it just comes down to restricting calories and increasing physical activity.

You can recognise a 'quick-fix' diet quite easily. If it sounds too good to be true it usually is. Avoid quick-fix diets that:

- Promise rapid weight loss
- Suggest that a particular food has magical fat-burning effects (e.g., grapefruit, lemon juice)
- Promote the avoidance of a whole food group or category of foods (e.g., starchy foods)
- Suggest eating mainly one type of food every day (e.g., cabbage soup)
- Don't address long-term changes to your eating habits and weight maintenance
- Don't recommend regular physical activity
- Don't warn people with a medical condition to seek medical advice.

Low-carbohydrate diets, e.g., The Atkins Diet

The humble carbohydrate has had a bad press recently, not all of which is deserved. Carbohydrates consist of sugars (confectionary, sugary drinks, table sugar, foods with added sugar) and starches (bread, pasta, rice, potatoes, chapatti and cereals).

Unless you are an elite athlete fuelling up after a run, it makes good common sense to limit sugary foods, as these contain largely 'empty calories' (energy with little additional nutrition). But starchy foods are better. They offer more nutrition and can be a source of valuable vitamins and minerals. As a good rule of thumb, the less processed the starchy food the more nutrition it contains. Wholegrains are packed full of nutrients as well as being a source of energy and they provide the best compromise. Not only are they rich in nutrients, but they also provide fibre to help satisfy appetite and help regulate and keep your bowels healthy.

Diets that advise over-restriction of starchy carbohydrates can put your health at risk. Your diet will simply be unbalanced. In particular, these types of diet restrict your intake of the essential B vitamins needed by your body to convert food into energy. Your intake of minerals such as potassium and magnesium will suffer too.

Many low-carbohydrate diets not only severely restrict carbohydrate foods; they may even limit your intake of fruits and vegetables. Meals are usually based on large portions of meat, fish, poultry and dairy products and typically encourage the use of liberal amounts of butter, oil, fatty meats and cream. During weight maintenance phases, the carbohydrate allowance is a little more relaxed but remains limited.

The emphasis on fat and protein means that these diets are usually rich in saturated fat. Not only are they not a good approach to weight loss, but they may even increase your cholesterol levels. While it is true some people do lose weight in the short term, this is only because the dietary rules mean that they unconsciously restrict their own energy intake. But such diets cannot be sustained over the long term without severe consequences for your nutrition, and they don't teach new and better eating habits. Side effects can include weakness, nausea, dehydration and bad breath.

Meal replacements

This approach can be appealing for a lot of people because of its simplicity. It involves replacing one or two meals each day with a meal replacement, such as a shake, cereal bar, soup or porridge, and preparing and eating a healthy meal in the evening.

Meal-replacement products are portion controlled, provide a known amount of energy and are usually fortified with extra vitamins and minerals to help ensure they provide the recommended amount of nutrients for good health.

It is possible to get bored with the meal-replacement products on offer after a while. But for many they take the pain out of planning an energy-restricted diet.

Weight-loss pills and potions

A variety of 'weight-loss products' are available over the Internet and at private clinics. Some of these may contain a form of soluble fibre that might have a modest effect on your appetite, but you will still need to exercise some control over the type of foods you eat and your portion sizes. Beware of products promising instant or unlikely levels of weight loss, especially if not openly advertised.

Any product that has been consistently shown to have a weight-loss effect will either be a medicine or will have been granted a health claim by the European Food Safety Authority. You can check online to see if this is the case.

Very Low Calorie Diets (VLCDs)

These are the most restrictive form of dieting where the daily calorie intake is severely reduced (800 kcalories or less), and for which medical supervision is generally recommended. VLCDs are scientifically proven to achieve effective weight loss and to be therapeutically effective in helping to treat certain conditions, such as sleep apnoea and osteoarthritis.

The foods that make up these diets are not usually available in shops and pharmacies but can be purchased through 'agents', who usually operate on a self-employed basis and have been trained to support people through their weight-loss journey. Companies include the Cambridge Weight Plan and Lighter Life. There are a range of calorie-restricted programmes, both weight loss and weight maintenance, from 400 to 1500 calories per day.

The VLCD foods are nutritionally balanced 'formula foods' designed to replace all meals. At least 2.25 litres of water (4 pints) must be taken in addition to the formula foods to help maintain normal hydration. Each programme comes complete with written information giving detailed instructions.

This approach could be helpful for very overweight people, especially when other approaches have not worked and where immediate weight loss is essential for medical reasons. Modest side effects can occur, such as headache, nausea, constipation, diarrhoea and dizziness, but these are usually because of insufficient water intake.

After the initial weight loss it is important to get support and advice in order to avoid rapid weight regain.

Surgery

Surgery to reduce stomach size (bariatric surgery) is only considered when all other approaches have been tried and have failed. The aim of the surgery is to make the stomach smaller either by using a 'gastric band' or by a gastric bypass. The result is that only small amounts of food can be eaten at any one time because you feel fuller after a lower food intake.

These approaches are only suitable for people who meet strict medical criteria and they require specialist aftercare and follow-up. Specialist dietary advice and support is needed to help adjust post-surgery and to ensure dietary intake is nutritionally balanced.

Slimming clubs

Slimming clubs have been around for many years and offer vital ongoing support as well as an opportunity for regular advice. Being in a supportive environment with other individuals who are also trying to lose weight can work well for many people, especially when the support of close family or friends is not available. Slimming clubs can be a helpful source of motivation, a forum for learning about and building new healthy habits, and for discussing your own needs.

There are a number of commercial slimming clubs such as Weight Watchers, Slimming World and Rosemary Conley. Meetings are weekly and weigh-ins happen in complete privacy. Confidentiality is guaranteed with no naming and shaming. In many cases the group leaders have successfully lost weight themselves, so they can understand and empathise with group members.

Most slimming clubs welcome men too. To find out what is on offer locally check online or ask at your local library, community centre or GP's surgery.

How are cholesterol levels affected by weight gain?

Modest increases in total and LDL-cholesterol levels often occur with weight gain. More worrying is that excess weight gain is linked to a condition known as insulin resistance. To explain this we need to know a bit more about insulin and what it does.

Insulin is an essential hormone that is produced in the pancreas by groups of cells called the islets of Langerhans that are scattered throughout the pancreas. Insulin has a number of functions in the body. Best known is its role in controlling the amount of sugars in the blood, but it also can affect the levels of circulating fats (cholesterol and triglycerides), and the lipo-proteins they are carried on, too. Insulin is vital for the use of sugar as an energy source in the body. It is also needed for normal growth.

'Insulin resistance' is the term given to describe a condition where the body's cells become resistant to the effects of insulin. It is usually a progressive condition that happens slowly and progresses over time. Gradually, usually over several years, the body's response to insulin is reduced so the pancreas has to produce more and more of it to compensate.

It might be helpful to think of insulin as a key that unlocks a door in the cell and allows sugar to be taken into the cell where it is used to produce energy. In insulin resistance the key doesn't work so well and more insulin has to be produced to open up the cell door to sugars.

As long as the pancreas is able to produce enough insulin, blood sugar levels remain normal. But there comes a point when the pancreas can no longer produce enough insulin for the body's needs. When this happens the amount of sugar in the blood rises. Initially this is only in the immediate period after meals but eventually sugar levels may be high all the time. When the amount of sugar in the blood rises above specific levels and fails to return to normal within a reasonable time frame diabetes is diagnosed.

Insulin resistance can also affect circulating blood fats

Insulin affects how the body manages dietary fat. It does this by stimulating the production of an enzyme called *lipoprotein lipase*. This enzyme is released into the blood where it sticks to the insides of tiny blood vessels called capillaries.

After a meal dietary fat is digested and enters the bloodstream as triglycerides. Under normal circumstances lipoprotein lipase acts on these triglycerides, and the lipoproteins that carry them (chylomicrons and VLDLs), breaking the triglycerides down into fatty acids. These fatty acids are either burnt for fuel or stored for later. The effect is a gradual removal of triglycerides from the circulation. Within a few hours of a meal, circulating triglyceride levels usually return to normal.

However in the case of insulin resistance, less lipoprotein lipase is produced. As a result circulating levels of triglycerides, and the lipoproteins that carry them, remain high.

Cholesterol levels can also increase with weight gain but the most significant effects on circulating blood fats are caused by insulin resistance. Below is a description of the typical effects of insulin resistance on blood fats and is characteristic of diabetes:

- Increased triglyceride levels (and circulating levels of chylomicrons and VLDLs)
- Decreased HDL cholesterol
- More smaller abnormal LDL-cholesterol particles.

Each of these characteristics (higher triglycerides, decreased HDL cholesterol, abnormal LDL particles) have been shown to increase the rate at which atherosclerosis – the furring up of blood vessels (see pages 37–42) – happens. So insulin resistance can play a central role in the development of cardiovascular disease.

The good news is that even modest reductions in weight loss and increased amounts of physical activity can improve the situation and so reduce cardiovascular risk.

Are you at risk of diabetes?

There are two types of diabetes. Type 1 diabetes usually develops in childhood and requires daily injections of insulin. Type 2 diabetes, however, usually but not always occurs in people who are overweight or obese. This is because with increasing weight gain the cells become less responsive to insulin. Because the cells are less responsive to insulin, the body begins to produce greater and greater amounts. In some people this increased production of insulin cannot be maintained, as the insulin-producing cells become exhausted. As a result, insulin levels decline and blood-sugar levels increase, eventually resulting in clinical diabetes.

Significant weight loss, resulting from reduced calorie intake and increased physical activity, can help to normalise blood-sugar levels in many, but for some medication, which helps to stimulate insulin production, is also necessary.

The number of people diagnosed with type 2 diabetes is increasing and it is believed that there are many more people with type 2 diabetes who remain undiagnosed.

Diabetes is also now recognised as a disorder of fat metabolism. This is because people with diabetes are less efficient at processing blood fats such as triglycerides and cholesterol.

In untreated, or in poorly controlled diabetics, a lack of insulin can lead to the release of large amounts of fatty acids from the fat stores and can also interfere with the activity of an enzyme (lipoprotein lipase – see page 68) which clears dietary fat from the blood after a meal.

Many people with type 2 diabetes (and pre-diabetes) share a common pattern of raised blood fats. This includes:

- Normal or slightly raised levels of cholesterol
- Moderately raised triglycerides
- Low-HDL cholesterol (good cholesterol)
- Smaller denser LDL cholesterol (bad cholesterol).

It is partly this distinctive pattern of altered blood fats that increases the risk of heart and circulatory disease in people with diabetes. Guidelines recommend that all adults with diabetes should have their blood fats measured and cardiovascular risk assessed every year.

Other factors (in diabetes) that increase cardiovascular disease risk include changes to the walls of blood vessels, which make them more vulnerable to developing atherosclerosis, and high blood pressure.

Because of the increased risk of cardiovascular disease, many people with diabetes are now routinely treated with a statin, especially if over the age of 40.

In Europe the lifetime risk of developing hyperglycaemia (raised blood sugar, a symptom of diabetes) is very high at around 80 per cent. The DECODE study has shown that during our lifetime 20 per cent of Europeans will be diagnosed as diabetics, 20 per cent will remain undiagnosed non-symptomatic diabetics, and a further 40 per cent will have some form of glucose intolerance (raised blood sugar not severe enough to merit a diagnosis of diabetes). Only

20 per cent will remain normoglycaemic (normal blood sugar) throughout our lifetimes.

The majority of us carry genes that permit diabetes to occur. Scientists in Canada and at Imperial College London recently announced they had identified several genes that explain up to 70 per cent of the inheritance factors. This important breakthrough could for the first time enable a genetic test to be developed which could help to identify those most at risk.

But diabetes is not inevitable. By making modest changes to our lifestyle, researchers believe we can reduce the risk of developing diabetes significantly, even in those with the early symptoms.

Summary

Obesity is a serious health problem that can affect your health and well-being.

Central obesity, or abdominal obesity:

- Increases the risk of cardiovascular disease
- Can cause insulin resistance which leads to an unhealthy pattern of blood fats (raised triglycerides and small dense LDL cholesterol, low-HDL cholesterol)
- Increases in blood sugar and ultimately the development of type 2 diabetes
- Can cause high blood pressure.

Small losses in weight if sustained can lead to marked improvements in blood pressure, blood lipids, and blood sugar control.

There are many methods of weight loss but it is important to:

- Start by assessing and making small changes to your own diet
- Both increase your activity and reduce your energy intake

- Set up support mechanisms among your friends, family and work colleagues, and enlist the advice of health professionals and slimming organisations
- Develop SMART aims and objectives for weight loss
- Learn from any relapses in eating behaviour and move forward from them.

PART 2

CHAPTER 5

How to lower cholesterol

N ow that you are more familiar with the science behind cholesterol and have a better understanding of how it might affect your health, you are ready to take action. The next four chapters will give you the insight, knowledge and practical, easy-to-follow strategies to help you lower your cholesterol levels. We know that making changes to your diet and lifestyle is not always easy so we have given you a simple step-by-step guide to help you achieve your goals.

The 4 key cholesterol-lowering steps

In this book we outline 4 key steps to improving your cholesterol levels. Each has an important role in reducing your risk of developing cardiovascular disease and preventing a heart attack or stroke.

Step 1: Motivation

Recognising the need for change, and being ready to make those changes, is central to reducing your cholesterol levels. So being motivated is the key to unlocking lifestyle change.

Step 2: Diet

Having a healthy diet is fundamental to lowering your cholesterol and helping to keep your heart healthy. A healthy diet has lots of other positive effects on your health too.

Step 3: Exercise and de-stress

Keeping physically active is essential at all times of life and doesn't necessarily mean having to go to the gym or joining a sports club. Giving your heart a little workout most days of the week helps to keep it in tip-top form. De-stressing is also part of step 3 and something many of us simply forget to do because we are so wrapped up in our busy hectic lives.

Step 4: Medication

Depending on the level of your LDL cholesterol and your overall cardiovascular risk, your doctor may or may not offer to treat your high cholesterol with medication from the very start. Usually doctors, lipid experts, nurses and dietitians will encourage you to try to make dietary and lifestyle changes first of all.

So the initial emphasis is on making small adjustments to the way you live your everyday life to help bring your cholesterol levels back towards normal as well as reduce your overall cardiovascular risk.

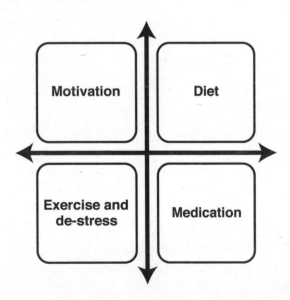

A word about smoking

While we don't include stopping smoking as one of our 4 steps to lowering cholesterol, we do recognise it is fundamental to managing your cardiovascular risk. Stopping smoking is the quickest way to improve your health, increase your protective HDL-cholesterol levels and lengthen your life expectancy. If stopping smoking is something you feel you can achieve, there is a lot of readily available expert support out there to help you. And it can be accessed easily too, just by searching online, picking up a leaflet at your library or GP surgery or by visiting your doctor or practice nurse.

Lifestyle change

Lifestyle change really is crucial to improving and maintaining good health, whether it is stopping smoking, being more physically active, managing stress levels or adopting a healthy diet: all have a role in helping to maintain good health and general well-being. Not only do they lower your risk of developing heart disease; they also help prevent many other chronic conditions such as weight gain, obesity, diabetes, respiratory and joint problems and cancer, as well as helping you feel good about yourself. Not only that but adopting healthy habits can have a positive effect on other family members too.

Most health professionals will advise you that it's not a case of choosing to make changes to your diet and lifestyle or choosing to take a medicine to lower your cholesterol. The two go hand in hand in helping to lower your risk. If you are offered a cholesterol-lowering drug and you decide to take it, it is **still** important to take care of your diet, be active and, if you smoke, to give it up. Your doctor won't ask you to tackle all these at once though.

Making lifestyle changes by yourself and adjusting to new healthier habits can be hard work. It's much easier if you involve other people around you who can provide support and encouragement, especially when the going gets tough.

Our first practical step is all about preparing yourself to make these changes. Being motivated and thinking through what you want to achieve and how to go about it are key to any kind of behaviour change, whether it is stopping smoking, losing weight or reducing your cholesterol.

There are some things that we know work well across all forms of behaviour change. Setting up a support mechanism, involving those around you and adopting a family-orientated approach to behaviour change mean you are more likely to succeed than if you set out to do it alone.

We wish you the very best on your own and your family's cholesterol-lowering journey. Let's get started!

CHAPTER 6

Step 1: Motivation

L ike most people, you've probably made promises to yourself to make healthier choices, begin exercising or quit smoking, and perhaps you've even stuck with these resolutions for a while. Too often, however, life gets in the way, and our best intentions fall by the wayside.

For most people, making a lifestyle change is not easy. Maintaining change is even harder, especially when making more than one change at the same time. In step 1 we have put together tips to help you plan to change, keep you motivated while you make the change and increase the likelihood of you reaching your health and wellness goals.

Changing behaviour is a process not an event. Everyone goes through five stages when changing any ingrained behaviour.

What are the five stages of change?

1. Pre-contemplation (not thinking about change)
Someone who is at the first stage is not really thinking about changing. They either like what they are doing or don't see it as a problem.

2. Contemplation (thinking about it, but not quite ready to change)
At this stage, someone is considering change but that is all they are doing. Although they are more aware of the consequences of what they are doing, they are not ready to change.

3. Preparation (getting ready to change)

If you are in the preparation stage, you have made the decision to change and are getting ready to make the change. This involves planning how to do it, even if it is only in your head.

4. Action (making change happen)

If you are in the action stage, you have begun to make some changes, perhaps using short-term rewards to keep you motivated.

5. Maintenance (keeping the change going)

If you are in the maintenance stage, you are keeping the changes going. The longer you are in this phase the more likely that the changes will become established habits. If you slip back or relapse you go back to a previous stage.

Where are you in the stages of behaviour change?

How ready are you to make lifestyle changes to manage your cholesterol? Which of these best describes you?

- **Thinking** about it but not quite ready to make any diet or lifestyle changes
- **Getting ready**: interested in and finding out about changes I could make to my diet and lifestyle
- **Making change happen**: following a cholesterol-lowering diet and getting regular exercise
- **Keeping the change going**: establishing new healthy habits.

There are always benefits and potential downsides to making changes in your daily life. Only when the benefits outweigh any negative aspects will you feel ready for action. Just reading this book suggests that you are at the contemplation or even the preparation stage.

To make change possible you must not only believe that you can make the change happen; you must work at making the changes too. Because your blood cholesterol is dependent on many factors, you will need to focus on more than one of these factors, but not all at once. Successful change only comes by being open to advice, deciding what is practical, committing to and making changes and regularly reviewing your own progress.

Try answering the following questions to see if you are ready to make some changes. Make some notes so you can refer back to these; it's a good motivational technique.

- Why do **YOU** want to lower your cholesterol levels?
- Why is it so important?
- What has kept you from making changes to your diet and lifestyle in the past?

Overcoming barriers to change

Barriers provide reasons for not making a change. They are different for each person but once you identify your barriers, you can develop strategies to overcome them and get on track to lowering your cholesterol.

The kinds of lifestyle barriers many people experience include the cost of making the behaviour change, time constraints, family pressures, not having the skills or knowledge to make the change and the temptation to stick or revert to your current lifestyle.

Cost

It's a common misconception that a healthy lifestyle has to be expensive. You do not have to enrol in a gym or buy expensive food items; there are plenty of inexpensive options available.

Simple ways to include more exercise that won't cost you money include walking or running outdoors, gardening, taking the stairs instead of the lift and parking the car further from your destination. Save money at the supermarket by buying fruits and vegetables on special offers or buying only those that are in season. Try local market stalls and traders; if you go later in the day you are more likely to pick up end-of-the-day bargains. Opt for supermarket own-brand canned, dried and frozen fruit and vegetables, including dried pulses and beans, to keep costs down. Replace some of the meat in stews and casseroles with beans, peas or pulses. Buy meat on special offer, two for the price of one, and freeze the other one for later use. Tinned oily fish like sardines and salmon is often cheaper than buying fresh, but they still contain heart-friendly omega-3 fats and have a long shelf life too. Use your leftovers. Leftover vegetables can go into soup, meat into stews, casseroles and stir-fries, and over-ripe fruit is perfect when blended to make a smoothie.

Time constraints

For many people, finding time to exercise and prepare healthy meals seems like an impossible challenge. However, with minor changes to your daily routine and a bit of pre-planning this too can be overcome. Consider squeezing in a brisk walk during your lunch break, or use the stairs instead of the lift at work. Park a bit further away from your normal parking place, or get off the bus a stop earlier. Save time on meal preparation by prepping multiple meals at once and keeping them in the freezer or refrigerator for quick and convenient meal options. Stock up on tinned, dried and frozen fruit and vegetables so you always have them ready to use.

Friends/family pressure

The social pressures to eat and drink, which come from family members, friends and work colleagues, may make it difficult to stick to your plan. Social events and interactions often revolve around food and, in many cases, alcohol consumption too, making it difficult to ignore the temptations around you. Although you might be tempted to keep your dietary goals to yourself, it can help to let your friends, family and colleagues know what you are trying to achieve and how important it is to you. Once they understand they are more likely to support and encourage you.

The barriers to achieving any goal can be overcome, so long as you are prepared to plan ahead. Knowing that you can reduce your risk of heart disease and stroke by lowering your blood cholesterol level can be a strong motivator.

Setting goals

Most people know what they should be doing for better health, but actually doing it gets difficult. Goal-setting is a powerful technique that can help you manage your blood cholesterol levels. At its simplest, the goal-setting process allows you to identify what success might look like.

You can have big and small goals but it is important to break any big goals down into small practical steps, each of which takes you a little way towards your overall goal of reducing your cholesterol. By knowing precisely what you want to achieve and setting smaller goals along the way, you are more likely to achieve your overall aim. Start by choosing two or three small changes. Small changes don't need to be difficult but their effects add up. Write yourself an action plan.

To help ensure your success make your goals **SMART** (Specific, Measureable, Attainable, Realistic and Time-orientated).

Specific: A specific goal has a much greater chance of being accomplished than a general goal. To make your goal specific you must answer the following questions:

- What do I want to achieve?
- What does success look like? Identify requirements and constraints.
- Why? List specific reasons, purpose or benefits of accomplishing the goal.

Example 1: A general goal would be, 'to lower my cholesterol'. But a specific goal would say, 'Lower my cholesterol by 15 per cent in three months by making changes to my diet and lifestyle'.

Example 2: A general food-based goal might be, 'to follow a cholesterol-lowering diet'. But a specific goal would be, 'to eat an oat-based breakfast cereal with skimmed milk five days a week'.

Measurable: This means to establish concrete criteria for measuring progress on each goal set. When you measure your progress, you stay on track and experience the exhilaration of achievement that can motivate you to reach your goals. To be measurable there must be some way of keeping track of what you are doing, for example, how many days you ate an oat-based cereal with skimmed milk or whether you achieved your ultimate goal of lowering cholesterol by 15 per cent in three months. Build in some measurements, such as the number of times you eat something each day of the week, the number of steps you might walk in a day, or the date when you will have changed specific behaviour. Track your progress so that you can feel good about your successes! Remember: even though your goal is to improve every week, some weeks will be better than others. Don't be discouraged when one week is not as good as the last. A few setbacks are normal and part of the process of change. Learn from any relapses and get back on track as quickly as you can.

Attainable: You should set goals that are slightly out of your immediate grasp but not so far out of your reach that you have no hope of achieving them. Setting goals you cannot hope to achieve is a real blow for your self-esteem. As you set goals, try to determine whether they are appropriate for your lifestyle. Can you still attain them even when you are busy or distracted? Don't over-commit and don't be afraid to fit your goals to your personal circumstances. For example, if you are trying to cut back on eating out, you may find it hard to suddenly prepare and eat all your meals and snacks at home. So start with at least one meal such as eating breakfast at home, instead of grabbing food from a café on your way to work. Reviewing your goals in this way helps to ensure they are achievable.

Realistic: To be realistic, a goal must represent a point that you are both willing and able to work towards. Don't aim too high. For example, if your goal is to lose weight, a weight loss of between 0.5–2 pounds a week is a safe and realistic target. Don't be tempted to set a target that you are unlikely to achieve without radically changing your habits or one that may compromise your health. Softly, softly is the best approach. You are also more likely to learn better habits by attempting gradual change over a longer time frame rather than looking for a quick fix that you cannot hope to maintain.

Time-orientated: Ground your goal within a time frame. With no time frame tied to it there's no sense of urgency. If you want to lose 5 kilograms, when do you want to lose it by? Don't forget to set a realistic time frame. If your goal might take you a long time to reach, set some smaller goals along the way, which will help keep you on track.

5 good reasons to set SMART goals:

- They help you focus
- They help you stay motivated
- They help you manage your time and effort
- They help you track your progress
- You are more likely to achieve them.

Goals often change as time moves on, and you should adjust your goals regularly to reflect your own personal growth and any new circumstances. The trick is being accountable to yourself (or being accountable to your support system of friends and family) to accomplish your SMART goal. Here are some examples of simple, cholesterol-lowering changes written as SMART goals:

Change: Switch to skimmed milk.
Why: Full-cream milk contains saturated fat, which can raise cholesterol levels.
How: Gradually wean yourself from the higher-fat varieties to the lower-fat milk. Your palate will fine-tune itself to the thinner, less creamy consistency of skimmed milk if you give it time to adjust.
Sample goal: I will switch to semi-skimmed (2 per cent fat) for one month. Then I will move to 1 per cent fat for a month. Finally, I will make the move to skimmed milk in the third month.

Change: Snack on a piece of fruit or a small handful of unsalted nuts instead of biscuits.
Why: Fruit and unsalted nuts are just as convenient as other typical snack foods and moreover the fibre, protein and good fats in nuts help keep hunger at bay and help lower cholesterol.
How: Keep a supply of fruit on your desk or nuts in your handbag or packed lunch, so if you are hungry or tempted by other snacks you have your preferred snack at hand.
Sample goal: I will swap my usual afternoon snack at work for a handful of unsalted nuts Monday to Friday for four weeks.

Change: Replace some meat with pulses.
Why: Pulses are not only low in fat and a very good source of soluble fibre but are also a good source of protein. Meat, especially fatty or processed meat, contains animal fat, a source of saturated fat.
How: Select one or more recipes where you can minimise the red meat content and add pulses to the dish, such as chilli con carne, casseroles, soups, salads and stir fries.

Sample goal: I will include pulses in two of my main meals each week as a way of either reducing or replacing red meat in these meals.

How to increase your chances of success

You can increase your chances of lowering your cholesterol by using the following strategies:

Get friends and family on board

A supportive atmosphere is important. If you are trying to live a healthier lifestyle and the rest of the family do not support you, you can feel isolated. This feeling of isolation can affect the amount of effort you put into managing your cholesterol. Eating is a highly social activity, whether you are eating with family, friends or colleagues, or celebrating a key event. By sharing your goals with others, you will move a step forward in enlisting their support. It is often easier to make lifestyle changes at the beginning when you are highly motivated, but as time goes on you will find it easier to stick to your resolve if you surround yourself with people who respect your goals and aspirations. Your support network can take different forms, such as people exercising with you, eating healthily together, or it may be asking about your progress, complimenting you on your success, or rewarding you when you do well.

Write it down

Write your goal down and post it somewhere you look often, like your bathroom mirror or fridge door. Keeping a food and activity diary can help you understand a lot about your eating and activity patterns, and highlight areas for change. (See chapter 7 for food diary.)

Reward yourself

Treat yourself when you achieve key points in your journey. Rewards serve to reinforce your behaviour change and provide a mental boost to help encourage you to carry on. Don't use food as your reward. Instead, treat yourself to a book or DVD or try rewarding yourself with extra time spent with a friend, a hobby you've wanted to pursue or an activity that keeps you moving. For example, take a dancing class for the first time with a friend or visit that special place you have always wanted to go to.

Review your successes and failures

When you achieve a goal, take the time to enjoy the satisfaction of achievement, give yourself a proper pat on the back. It is important to review when you have failed to reach a goal too. Reviewing what went wrong gives you greater self-knowledge and helps you plan how to achieve your next goal. If you are finding your goals are easily achieved, make your next goal harder. If the goal took a dispiriting amount of effort or time to achieve, make the next goal a little easier.

Change your routine

Routine can be the biggest killer of motivation. You need to change it to stay excited about what you are doing. If you use the same route for a walk day after day, change your routine by walking somewhere else. Don't eat the same things for breakfast, lunch and dinner every week. Try new dishes. Look for alternative healthy options. Variety is the spice of life!

Get professional help

Changing your lifestyle can seem overwhelming, even when you know to make only one or two changes at a time. Ask your doctor to refer you to see a registered dietitian for nutritional counselling or to an exercise scheme. Make the most of any help offered by your doctor's surgery. Think through what you want to achieve and any questions you might want to ask before any appointment. Getting professional support not only helps keep you inspired but can help you through tough times too.

Setting goals to help lower your cholesterol

- Determine your stage of readiness to change
- Decide on your overall goal – what do you want to achieve and by when
- Identify barriers you face and develop strategies to avoid or overcome these barriers
- Set goals for eating, physical activity and other areas of your lifestyle making sure they re specific, measurable, attainable, realistic, and time-oriented
- Review your progress regularly to help motivate and improve.

Preventing Relapses

Relapses can happen at any time. It's quite normal to have times when you slip up and are tempted back to a less healthy lifestyle. Temptations strike fast and hard. Before you know it, you've eaten that large packet of crisps meant for sharing. When this happens:

Stay positive

Having a positive approach will help you put this temporary lapse behind you and move on. Say to yourself, 'Eating the whole packet doesn't mean I've blown it. I'm in control and am back on track.' Resist any negative self-talk as it is likely to mean your lapse will become a complete relapse. So avoid thinking, 'I've just eaten that big packet and blown all my good intentions. I might as well forget the cholesterol-lowering diet and eat what I want now,' and instead accept that the occasional slip up is normal and it's not the end of the world. Get straight back on track. Don't let a slip make you lose sight of your overall goals and the good progress you have made.

Cause of lapse

Think about what caused the lapse. Peer pressure? Bored? Too busy? Have a plan for your high-risk situations. So if you know you are more likely to slip up when you are busy, plan ahead to handle this situation. For example, write weekly meal plans, write shopping lists, cook in bulk and freeze individual portions.

Keep a food diary

This may not stop you eating unhealthy foods altogether, but it could keep you from acting on a whim. For example, the thought of writing down the meat pie you are craving may just stop you eating it. A food diary will also help you identify the times and situations in the day when the temptation to eat unhealthy foods is strongest. (See page 146 for how to keep a food diary.)

Plan for events such as eating out, celebrations and parties

Having the odd unhealthy meal is unlikely to make a difference to your cholesterol levels in the long run, but these days we eat out far more than ever before. Decide what your plan of action will be and stick to it. For example, when eating out, decide to have two courses instead of three. Share a starter or a pudding rather than having your own. When you are with a group, be the first to order so you are not swayed by others ordering less healthy choices.

Eat a varied diet

Eating the same foods every day may leave you feeling unfulfilled. Be creative in the kitchen, try combining different tastes and textures and experiment with new foods.

Keep it in the family

The family plays a vital and important role in influencing a child's health behaviours, such as eating habits, smoking, drinking and physical activity. Parents set the stage for positive and negative behaviours within the household and are the primary role models for their children. Remember: actions speak louder than words. It's no good saying 'do this' or 'do that' when your own behaviour does not reflect the verbal messages you are giving your child.

The bottom line is that a parent's attitude towards their own health can strongly affect their child's attitude too. Are there improvements to be made to your family's lifestyle and eating habits? The same rules apply. Aim for small achievable steps.

When it comes to children there are so many ways you can make a difference, such as encouraging them in active play, developing a liking for sport, family bike rides, walks and outings, trips to the park, walking the dog, walking part or all the way to school and back, learning to cook, growing their own food, trying new foods, limiting sweets and swapping sugary drinks for water.

Set SMART goals to inspire change.

Remember there is no quick fix. People who successfully make changes to their diets and maintain these changes stay realistic and develop techniques to make their new lifestyle and activity habits an enjoyable way of life.

Summary

- Start by deciding what stage of change you are in. Are you ready to make a change? If not, why not? What might move you to the next stage?
- Decide on your overall goal and break it down into small and manageable steps. Write an action plan. Make sure your goals are SMART.
- Set up your support network, monitor your progress, reward yourself and readjust your goals if necessary.
- Don't give up, even if it gets tough or you relapse, identify patterns of problem behaviour and ways of getting around the problem.

CHAPTER 7

Step 2: Diet

C hanging your eating habits is one of the most effective ways to improve your cholesterol. By eating more healthily, your body will enjoy a range of benefits, including: reaching and keeping a healthier weight; safeguarding your vitamin and mineral intake, which is vital for the normal functioning of our bodies; improved blood sugar control if you are diabetic; more energy and fewer problems such as bloating or constipation. In this section, we'll dispel some of the myths around food types and provide a clear, heart-healthy road map for what to eat and what to avoid.

Following our recommendations doesn't mean starving yourself and you will still be able to enjoy a wide variety of foods. In particular it is important to fill up on heart-healthy foods that are low in calories yet still satisfying.

General guidelines to remember:

- About a third of your food should be carbohydrate-rich foods such as bread, potatoes, chapattis, pasta, rice and other cereals. These foods do not contain too many calories unless you add fat to them.
- Most of us eat too little fibre, so where possible try to choose wholemeal or wholegrain varieties. Wholegrains also contain higher levels of nutrients and are more satisfying than refined carbohydrates such as sugars and white bread.
- Eat plenty of vegetables, salads and fruit. At mealtimes try to cover half of your plate with vegetables. Fresh, canned, frozen

and dried fruit and vegetables all count, but if choosing canned fruit go for those in natural juices rather than syrup.

• Try increasing your intake of pulses, beans, peas and lentils. These are all low in calories but high in fibre so are excellent choices.

How to change your diet

This chapter is divided into two key parts and it's best to work through it in stages. The first part focuses on adopting a cardio-protective way of eating. This is something we all should do whether or not our cholesterol is high.

We recommend fully adopting the cardio-protective diet first before progressing further. It is based on good nutritional principles and forms the foundation for the second part of this chapter. These initial changes may be easy for some and more difficult for others; but it is likely that everyone will see some reduction in their cholesterol levels as a result. The more changes you make to your diet to reflect the cardio-protective diet, the more impact it will have on your cholesterol levels.

The second part of this chapter is dedicated to some key foods and food groups that when eaten in significant quantities can help to lower your cholesterol further. We call them 'cholesterol busters'. Some of these already form a part of the cardio-protective diet, however, in the latter part of this chapter we go on to describe exactly how you can optimise your cholesterol lowering by including them on a daily basis. It is this combination of the cardio-protective diet and the cholesterol busters that provides the biggest potential for cholesterol reduction through lifestyle change.

Stage 1: The cardio-protective diet

Welcome to Stage 1 of transforming your diet. The cardio-protective diet is the name given to a Mediterranean style of eating that has been shown to protect our hearts. This regular way of eating is recommended for everyone looking to maintain a healthy heart, regardless of their cholesterol levels. Because it is suitable for both children and adults it is a great way to feed the family.

We know this way of eating is protective because of the work of some clever researchers. Even as early as the 1960s, Dr Ancel Keys, a pioneering American epidemiologist, and his colleagues examined the relationship between diet and heart disease rates in seven countries. The study found that people who lived along the Mediterranean Sea had much lower rates of heart attacks and death from heart disease compared to those living in the more industrialised parts of Europe. The population of Greece, and in particular people from the island of Crete, had the lowest rates of death from heart disease and the longest life expectancy. A Cretan diet is rich in legumes, fruits, vegetables, olive oil and red wine. The diet is also high in the essential omega-3 fatty acid – alpha-linolenic acid (see pages 115–16) and much lower in the omega-6 essential fatty acid linoleic acid (see pages 115–16) than other Mediterranean diets.

The cardio-protective diet originates from Ancel Keys' initial research and continues to be acclaimed to this day following further extensive investigation. Why does it work so well? Simply because a cardio-protective way of eating has been shown to help maintain heart health and reduce the risk of CVD in several ways. The first of these is by helping to lower LDL-cholesterol levels.

The second is by helping to reduce the background inflammation in the body. This means lowering the sensitivity of the linings of the blood vessel walls (the endothelium) and improving its ability to defend against the entry of cholesterol.

The cardio-protective diet also plays a role in helping to maintain normal blood sugar levels and blood pressure, two significant risk factors for CVD. The key elements of the cardio-protective diet are explained in the following pages.

Fruit and vegetables

Aim to eat **at least** five portions (about 400 g) of vegetables and fruit each day. Fresh, frozen, dried, canned and pure juices all count. The only exceptions are potatoes, yams and cassava, which are starchy foods and so are not included in the recommended five-a-day. Also, no matter how much you drink, a glass of juice only counts as one portion. The reason that juice only counts once is that it is a more processed form of fruit and the valuable fibre from the fruit is removed. This makes juice very easy to drink in large quantities without necessarily satisfying your appetite. It's important to remember that a glass of juice can contain as much as 4–5 teaspoons of sugar in just one 150 ml serving.

Choose a variety of fruits and vegetables over the day to benefit from all the different vitamins and minerals and cardio-protective nutrients they contain. Nutrients, such as vitamin C, beta carotene, folic acid, vitamin E, zinc and selenium, all help protect the body from damaging free radicals, which in large quantities can cause cell damage.

As a guide, the more colourful your plate, the greater the variety of nutrients you get. In addition, many fruits and vegetables are good sources of phytochemicals, naturally occurring plant chemicals that are also powerful antioxidants. Examples are the flavonoids. Flavonoids are found in many different foods, especially apples, tea and onions. As well as helping to reduce the levels of harmful free radicals, research also suggests that flavonoids may help to make the blood less sticky, therefore potentially reducing the chances of harmful blood clots (thrombosis).

In addition all fruits and vegetables are a good source of fibre. High intakes of dietary fibre have been associated with a reduced risk of heart disease as well as some cancers. Soluble fibre (see page 127) found in pulses (beans, peas and lentils) and some fruits (such as apples, strawberries and prunes) and vegetables (such as aubergine, broccoli, sweet potato, okra) can play a role in helping to reduce cholesterol levels.

What counts as a portion?

An adult portion of fresh, canned or frozen fruit or vegetables is 80 g (3 oz).

- 1 whole fresh fruit e.g., apple, pear, orange, banana, peach
- 3 heaped tablespoons of vegetables, beans or pulses*
- 1 dessert bowl of salad
- 2 medium fruits, e.g. plums, apricots, satsumas, kiwi fruits
- 1 slice of large fruits e.g., melon, pineapple
- a handful of small fruits e.g., grapes, berries, cherries, lychees
- 3 heaped tablespoons of tinned fruit in natural juice
- 3 heaped tablespoons of stewed fruit
- Dried fruit or vegetables – 1 heaped tablespoon
- Fruit or vegetable juice – 150 ml (1/4 pint) pure fruit or vegetable juice.

Smoothies, containing all the edible fruit, may contribute to more than one portion depending on the quantity. To qualify as two portions a smoothie has to contain the equivalent of two different 80 g portions of whole fruit and vegetables OR one 80 g portion of whole fruit or vegetable and 150 ml of a different pure fruit or vegetable juice.

Don't forget to count the vegetables you add to cooked dishes, for example, onions or mushrooms in stews and casseroles, tomatoes in a pasta sauce, or dried fruit in breakfast cereals.

Dairy products, meat and fish

Dairy products

Traditionally high in fat, milk, cheese, yoghurt and butter were all eaten in fairly small quantities in a traditional Mediterranean

---

*Beans/pulses count as a maximum of one portion of vegetables per day due to their lower micronutrient content compared to other fruit and vegetables. However, they are an excellent source of soluble fibre and protein.

diet. As well as our main source of calcium, which is essential for healthy bones, milk and dairy foods also provide us with protein and vitamins A and B$_{12}$. Because they are highly nutritious it's best not to cut them out of the diet completely unless you replace them with equivalent plant-based foods, such as fortified soya milk and soya-based desserts.

If you do stick to dairy then make sure you choose the lower-fat options such as semi-skimmed, 1 per cent fat or skimmed milk, low-fat yoghurts and half-fat hard cheeses or lower-fat soft cheeses. Low-fat dairy foods still contain the same amount of protein and calcium as their full-fat counterparts but significantly lower total and saturated fat. When you remove the fat from dairy foods you also remove the vitamin A, a fat-soluble vitamin. Provided your diet is rich in fruits and vegetables, you don't need to worry because dark green, orange and yellow fruits and vegetables provide a source of beta carotene from which our bodies can naturally make vitamin A.

It is important to have at least two or three portions of dairy foods each day to help ensure an adequate intake of calcium. Growing teenagers may need up to four portions. A typical portion is a 200 ml glass of milk, 150 g pot of yoghurt, two tablespoons of cottage cheese or a matchbox-sized piece of cheese. Tofu, calcium-fortified soya milks and juices, sesame seeds, the bones of canned fish, green leafy vegetables and hard tap water are all good non-dairy calcium sources.

Meat and fish

The Western style of eating is based around large portions of meat at the centre of the meal, with vegetables and starchy foods as accompaniments. As a result, most of us eat more meat than is necessary to maintain health. Think of the meat or fish as more of a flavour accompaniment to your main meal of starchy wholegrains and vegetables or salad.

A portion of meat, when cooked, should be approximately the same size as a deck of cards and fish should be the size of a chequebook. A grilled pork chop (without fat, rind or crackling), a chicken breast, two to three slices of roast meat or a fillet of fish are examples of the portion size to aim for. Choose red meats just two to three times a week and processed meats, such as ham, bacon or sausages, even less frequently as they are usually high in saturated fat and salt. In total you should limit your combined intake of red and processed meat each week to no more than 500g cooked weight, 700–750 g raw weight.

Choosing lean cuts of meat and trimming off any visible fat helps to reduce the saturated fat content further. Chicken, turkey and many game meats are lower in fat than most red meat, but do not eat the skin which is the fattiest part. Goose and duck are rich in saturated fat so keep these for special occasions.

White fish is an excellent source of protein and is low in fat. Try to include some oily fish (see page 116) at least once a week as the omega-3 fatty acids found in oily fish are excellent for heart health (see page 116).

Vegetable sources of omega-3 include green leafy vegetables, especially broccoli, spinach or cabbage; soya or rapeseed oils, walnuts, flaxseeds (linseeds) and their oils and foods fortified with omega-3.

Fats

A cardio-protective diet is low in saturated fat. Animal fats like butter, lard and ghee (clarified butter) are little used in the traditional Mediterranean diet. That's because olive oil, grown in abundance in Mediterranean countries, is the main source of fat. Olive oil produced in the first pressing is called extra virgin olive oil. This first pressing contains phenolic compounds, which provide its unique aroma and taste and are believed to provide additional cardiovascular health benefits. They act as antioxidants, which help to mop up dangerous chemicals called 'free radicals' which come from being exposed to chemicals in pollution, food and cigarette smoke. Free radicals can damage cell walls, DNA and the inside wall of blood vessels. They can also make LDL cholesterol more sticky and more likely to infiltrate the blood vessel wall.

A large proportion of these fragile phenolic compounds are lost when the oil is heated so, although you can cook with them, it's best to save extra virgin oils for salad dressings.

Most vegetable oils are extracted from seeds by solvents, whereas olive oil is obtained from the whole fruit by means of physical pressure, without the use of chemicals. Rapeseed oil (known as canola oil in North America) is a good alternative. It is produced from the rapeseed plant, which is the third most important crop in the UK. Its neutral taste is preferred by some to the strong taste of olive oil, and its 10 per cent omega-3 content makes it a useful alternative. Remember that every tablespoon of oil contains 135 kcals, so if you are trying to lose weight, only use modest amounts of whichever oil you choose. We talk in more detail about reducing saturated fat intake later in this chapter. It is not only important to lower saturated fat; it is fundamental to replace this fat with heart-healthy unsaturated fats in order to fully reflect the pattern of eating in the Mediterranean. The Mediterranean diet is not a low-fat diet; the emphasis is on having more of the healthy unsaturated fats and less saturated fats: in other words, more seeds, nuts and oils and less butter, ghee and lard.

Wholegrain breads, cereals, nuts and legumes

People living in Mediterranean countries tend to consume a wide variety of cereals, grains and other starchy foods. Staple foods in this region include bread, pasta, rice, oats, bulgur wheat, tabbouleh, couscous, semolina, gnocchi and potatoes.

About a third of your plate should be made up of starchy wholegrain foods. This food group should provide around half of all your energy requirements, along with a good proportion of the vitamins and minerals your body needs and small amounts of protein too. Aim to include one food from this group at each mealtime, choosing wholegrain varieties whenever possible.

Wholegrains such as wheat, corn, barley, oats and rye provide important cardio-protective nutrients such as the B group vitamins, vitamin E, zinc and selenium. These nutrients along with their beneficial levels of dietary fibre confer the positive health benefits of wholegrains. Many health experts now recommend eating three servings of wholegrains every day.

Examples of some wholegrain foods and portion sizes

Type of food	Wholegrain varieties	Amount needed to provide 1 wholegrain serving
Breakfast cereal	Whole oats including rolled oats and oatmeal, wholewheat cereals such as Weetabix, Shreddies, Shredded wheat, Bran Flakes etc.	2 heaped tablespoons uncooked oats or wholegrain cereal, I wholegrain breakfast biscuit
Bread and crackers	Wholemeal, granary or rye bread, wholemeal pitta, whole wheat crackers, oatcakes and rye crispbread	One medium slice bread ½ wholemeal pitta 2 rye crispbreads 2 oatcakes or whole wheat crackers
Flour	Wholemeal, wheat germ, barley, buckwheat, oatmeal, oat flour	20 g flour
Meals	Brown rice, whole wheat pasta, bulgur wheat, quinoa, whole barley	55–60 g cooked weight (e.g., 2 heaped tablespoons cooked brown rice or 3 tablespoons wholegrain pasta) 80 g (cooked weight) quinoa
Snacks	Wholegrain cereal bars or scone, wholegrain rice cakes, popcorn (plain)	1 small cereal bar 1 small scone (35 g) 2–3 cups plain popcorn (30 g)

A note on sugar-sweetened cereals

Sugar and health

To date there has been very little evidence demonstrating that sugars added to the diet have any direct effect on cholesterol levels or cardiovascular disease. There is however evidence to show that frequent consumption of sugars in the form of sugary drinks and confectionary can cause tooth decay. Excess consumption of sugars can also lead to increased energy intake, weight gain and an increase in BMI. There is also limited evidence of a relationship between sugar intake and the incidence of type 2 diabetes, but admittedly further good-quality research needs to be conducted in this area.

Lots of foods contain sugar. Of course it is possible to cut all refined sugar out of your diet, but in reality it is neither necessary, nor practical. The UK dietary recommendations for healthy eating recommend that no more than 10 per cent of our calorie intake should come from added sugars but this is under review; an eminent scientific body recently called to reduce this to just 5 per cent. This includes table sugar, confectionary, sugary drinks, honey, preserves like jam and marmalade, and that added to foods during cooking, manufacture or processing. It does not include sugar in fruit (where it is still encapsulated within the cellular structure of the fruit) or milk sugars. However, when you look at food packaging, the reference to the sugar content is to all sugars as it is impossible to discriminate analytically between intrinsic sugars (those in fruit and milk) and extrinsic or added sugars. So when trying to limit sugar it is best to bear the following tips in mind:

- Cut down on foods and drinks that contain sugar but very little else. This includes sugar-sweetened beverages like fizzy soft drinks and cordials, sweets and other confectionary and table sugars. It is also a good idea to limit cakes, biscuits and puddings.
- Sugars naturally present in other foods pose fewer problems, mainly because they come alongside other nutrients that are beneficial to us. Examples are the sugar in an orange or the sugar in fromage frais or yoghurt.

- Sugar can help make foods palatable, such as breakfast cereals and low-fat yoghurts. Without the sugar (naturally derived or not) these foods will fail to appeal to most people. In fact many people who buy unsweetened breakfast cereals or porridge actually add sugar or honey to it to improve the taste, perhaps adding more than the manufacturer would.
- When sugars are present in wholefoods like fruit and in complex foods like wholegrain breakfast cereals this sugar is absorbed slowly and raises blood sugar much more gently than sugars in sweetened drinks, table sugar and even white bread.
- If you are going to eat or drink something very sugary, the effects on your blood sugar and oral health can be dampened down by having it alongside a healthy meal. The meal helps to buffer the effect – hence the advice to parents to keep sweet treats to after mealtimes.

Starchy wholegrain foods are a source of both insoluble and soluble fibre. Insoluble fibre, found in the outer layer of wholegrains, is important for improving bowel function and preventing constipation. Soluble fibre, mainly found in oats, barley and rye, works to slow down the digestion of foods, helping to regulate appetite, improve blood sugar levels and reduce LDL cholesterol (see page 127.)

Legumes, such as beans, peas and pulses are good sources of both insoluble fibre and the cholesterol-lowering soluble fibre and are full of cardio-protective nutrients such as arginine, vitamin E, the B vitamins and minerals. They are naturally low in fat and are a useful source of protein that can replace or extend meat or fish dishes. The great selection of canned beans and pulses available in most stores means you no longer have to soak and boil legumes, and makes it easy to incorporate them into many recipes.

Alcohol

Alcohol is a small but significant feature of the Mediterranean diet. A daily intake of 1 to 2 units of alcohol is associated with lower risk of CHD in men aged over 40–45 and in women who have been through the menopause. Scientists believe there are two main mechanisms by which alcohol can help in CHD prevention. The main effect is an increase in high-density lipoprotein (HDL). Secondly, moderate alcohol intake may help prevent the formation of blood clots, reducing the level of fibrinogen, a protein that is produced by the liver and increases the likelihood of blood clotting. Other components of alcoholic drinks may provide further protection such as flavonoids found in red wine. This is still not conclusive and more research is needed to demonstrate the cardio-protective benefits of red wine over other forms of alcohol. Drinking alcohol with meals may be more beneficial to health than drinking it on its own.

The benefits of alcohol are quickly lost at higher intakes. People who persistently exceed the sensible drinking limits are more likely to suffer from conditions such as high blood pressure, which increases the risk of having a heart attack or stroke (see page 28), some types of cancer, reduced fertility and liver problems. Binge drinking may also cause abnormal heart rhythms, and regular heavy drinking can enlarge the heart, or cause damage to a developing baby during pregnancy.

Gaining weight and an increase in waist circumference (both risk factors for CHD, see page 55) can also result from drinking excess alcohol. One unit of alcohol contains 8 g or 10 ml of alcohol, which provides 56 kcals. Therefore a large glass of wine (250 ml) can add over 220 kcals to your meal. Drink 2–3 units a day and you could consume 6,000 calories a month!

Over-consumption of alcohol is also associated with increased levels of triglycerides in the blood. (see page 47)

Recommended safe limits

A safe upper limit of alcohol intake for a man is 3–4 units a day with at least two alcohol-free days. For women, a safe upper limit is 2–3 units of alcohol a day with the same alcohol-free days as men. Be aware that having alcohol-free days does not mean increasing the amounts drunk on other days!

What is a unit?

A unit is a measure of alcohol. The number of units in a drink is based on the size of the drink and its alcohol strength. The ABV (alcohol by volume) figure is the percentage of alcohol in the drink. Most drinks declare their ABV on the label.

1 unit of alcohol:

- 1 single pub measure (25 ml) of spirits (ABV 40 %)
- ½ pint (about 300 ml) of normal-strength lager, cider or beer (3.5% ABV)
- 1 small glass (100 ml) of wine (10% ABV)
- 1 glass (50 ml) of liqueur, sherry or other fortified wine (ABV 20%).

Keep an eye on your glass size! A standard small glass of wine in a pub is actually 175 ml, so that would be 2 units of alcohol if you are drinking a 12% ABV wine.

To work out the number of units in a drink multiply the % ABV by the amount of drink in millilitres. Then divide by 1000.

For example, to calculate the number of units in a 300 ml can of beer (5% ABV)

$$= 300 \times 5 \div 1000$$
$$= 1500 \div 1000$$
$$= 1.5 \text{ units of alcohol}$$

Many websites provide drink calculators to help you work this out.

Alcohol and medicines

It may be necessary to avoid alcohol if you are taking certain medicines. Ask your doctor or pharmacist if you are unsure about drinking alcohol with any medicines you are taking, or check the patient information leaflet that comes with your medication. There are no known interactions between statins and alcohol but it is important to stay within safe guidelines.

Alcohol and pregnancy

All health experts advise women who are pregnant, breastfeeding or trying to conceive to stop drinking altogether in order to protect the developing baby. Alcohol can pass through the placenta to the developing baby, who is less able to deal with it than adults. Even moderate drinking could cause harm, especially early in pregnancy.

Adopting the Mediterranean style of eating will help you to lower your risk of heart disease and stroke. However, if you think attempting to take on the whole plan in one go may be over-ambitious, why not try addressing one new aspect each week? (See pages 82–91 on setting achievable goals).

A balanced approach is the best. You can still enjoy the odd indulgence from time to time, provided that the majority of the time you follow the eating plan. Remember the cardio-protective diet is just part of a whole lifestyle approach towards better heart health. Not smoking and taking plenty of physical activity (see pages 155–7) are also part of this lifestyle package.

Summary

A cardio-protective diet:

- Is rich in fruits, vegetables, legumes (beans, peas, pulses), wholegrain cereals, seeds and nuts and the cardio-protective nutrients they contain
- Is low in saturated fat from dairy and meat sources
- Uses olive oil (an unsaturated fat) as the main fat for cooking and salad dressings
- Includes a variety of seafood and other non-meat proteins such as nuts
- Contains alcohol, but in modest amounts.

Getting the fats right

Fats (which includes both solid fats and liquid oils) are an important part of our diet as they provide us with around a third of our energy. We naturally store fat beneath the skin (subcutaneous fat) and around our organs (visceral fat) to be called upon when food intake is limited. Our fat stores also provide insulation against the cold and some protection to our organs. Fats and oils are also carriers of the fat-soluble vitamins A, D, E, and K and provide a source of the essential fats, linoleic acid and alpha-linolenic acid. These essential fats and fat-soluble vitamins cannot be made in the body so it is essential we have a supply in our diet.

While a heart-healthy diet is **NOT** a low-fat diet, it is important to be aware that eating too much fat can make us more likely to become overweight because fat is a concentrated source of calories, providing nine calories per gram – that's more than double the four calories per gram from carbohydrates (sugars and starches) or protein (see page 57). About a third of your energy should come from fats. An average man requires around 2,500 calories (kcals) per day; an average woman 2,000 calories (kcals) per day. For most men that means no more than 90–95 g of fat and women no more than 70–75 g fat per day.

Different types of fat

There are four main types of fat in our diet. Some fats are better for our health than others. Fats that are considered to be less healthy, because they can raise our blood cholesterol levels, are saturated fats and trans fats. Replacing these fats with unsaturated fats helps to lower cholesterol.

Healthy fats

- Monounsaturated fat
- Polyunsaturated fat

Unhealthy fats

- Saturated fat
- Trans fat

Most foods are a complex mixture of proteins, fats, carbohydrates, vitamins and minerals. Basic foods such as meat, fish, eggs, seeds, nuts, cereals and dairy foods all contain fats. But it is not quite that simple. Each of these foods contains a mixture of different fats from the list above. The trick is to know which foods contain more of the healthy fats and which more of the unhealthy fats. Generally speaking, animal fats (found in meat, dairy foods, butter, lard, ghee) tend to have higher levels of saturated fat; seafood, cereals, nuts and seeds tend to contain more of the healthy fats. There are two exceptions: palm oil, a common ingredient in processed foods, and coconut oil, often promoted as a health food, are mainly composed of saturated fats. Coconut oil contains around 85–90 per cent saturated fat.

Oils and fats are often spoken of as saturated, monounsaturated or polyunsaturated if they are mainly composed of one of these types of fat. Olive oil, for example, is classified as a monounsaturated fat even though it contains some saturated and polyunsaturated fat. This is because three-quarters of its fat is monounsaturated. Food labels often give the type of fat present in the food, as well as the amount. (See pages 132–6 on food labels.)

Example of how fats are described in the nutrition information panel of food packets

	Typical values	Typical values
	Per 100 g	Per 25 g serving
Fat	32.1 g	8.0 g
Of which saturates	2.6 g	0.7 g
Of which monounsaturates	25.3 g	6.3 g
Of which polyunsaturates	4.2 g	1.0 g

What are the differences between saturated and unsaturated fats?

All fats are made up of atoms of carbon and hydrogen joined together in a chain. They have a central spine, which is made up of carbon. Some fats have a short carbon chain (4–8 carbons), some medium (10–16 carbons) and others have a long carbon chain (18–22+ carbons long). All fats have an acidic group (COOH) at one end and a methyl group (CH_3) at the other end of their chain; this is why they are often referred to as fatty acids. Here are some examples of saturated and unsaturated fatty acids.

The carbon chains of different fats

Saturated fatty acid (stearic acid)

Monounsaturated fatty acid (oleic acid)

Polyunsaturated fatty acid
(linolenic acid–an omega-3 fatty acid)

Saturated fats get their name because they are saturated with hydrogen atoms. This means every carbon has the maximum number of hydrogen atoms bound to it and all their bonds are single bonds. This makes saturated fats very stable. They are also straight and rigid and can be tightly packed together to form solids. Hence saturated fats are usually solid at room temperature, such as butter or lard or the fat on meat.

Unsaturated fats differ because they have one or more double bonds and this makes the chain curve. The more double bonds, the more curved their shape. This means they cannot pack closely together, hence unsaturated fats are usually liquid at room temperature.

Monounsaturated fats have a single double bond; polyunsaturated fats have two or more double bonds.

Unsaturated fats are often described by the position of their first double bond. Omega-3, –6 and –9 fatty acids have their first double bond on the third, sixth and ninth carbon respectively.

Double bonds in Omega-3 and Omega-6 fatty acids

Saturated fat

Saturated fats have a major influence on the amount of cholesterol in the blood. They are usually solid at room temperature and generally of animal origin.

Foods that contain mainly saturated fats include:

- Butter, ghee, lard, hard margarines and foods made from these (cakes, biscuits, puddings, pies, pastries and pasties)
- Dairy produce (full-cream milk, cheese, full-fat yoghurt, crème fraîche and cream)
- Fatty meats and meat products (sausages, burgers, salami)
- Palm and coconut oils.

It is generally thought that reducing saturated fat intake can reduce LDL (bad) cholesterol by around 5–10 per cent. But the true effect is really based on how much change people are able to make. Someone who is already eating a relatively healthy diet may not be able to reduce their saturated intake much further. In the UK our dietary guidelines recommend lowering saturated fat intake to less than 10 per cent of our total energy intake or less than a third of our total fat intake.

Guideline intakes for fat and saturated fat

	Energy intake in calories	Total fat in grams	Saturated fat in grams
Average man	2,500	No more than 95 g	No more than 30 g
Average woman	2,000	No more than 70 g	No more than 20 g

Trans fats (partially hydrogenated vegetable oils)

Trans fats are found naturally in small amounts in meat and dairy products but they are also formed when vegetable oils undergo partial hydrogenation, an industrial process that hardens liquid oils to improve their storage qualities and to change their cooking properties. Fully hydrogenated oils are saturated fats; but partial hydrogenation produces trans fats, which are considered even more harmful. Trans fats that occur naturally don't appear to be harmful to our health, although there is still some debate surrounding this issue.

Man-made trans fats raise LDL (bad) cholesterol and lower HDL (good) cholesterol levels. This double effect makes trans fats the least desirable of all the fats, so avoid foods with trans fats whenever possible. Due to their harmful effects, much of the UK food industry has voluntarily removed them from the food chain. It is recommended that we eat less than 2 per cent of our energy as trans fats and average intakes are now about half of this.

The main sources of industrially produced trans fat are cakes, pastries, ready meals, deep-fried foods and biscuits. Manufacturers are not required to declare the amount of trans fat in their products, so you won't see this information under the nutritional information panel on foods. However, they should be declared as part of the ingredient list. See the box below for an example.

Ingredients: wheat flour, *partially hydrogenated vegetable oil*, sugar, glucose, eggs

Healthy fats

Unsaturated fats can play a big part in helping to keep us healthy. Not only are they are necessary for normal growth and development but increasing evidence suggests that unsaturated fats can play a role in improving cholesterol levels, preventing cardiovascular disease, improving our circulation, reducing blood clotting and reducing inflammation in our joints.

This is not an invitation to eat fats in unlimited quantities however. A careful balance of healthier fats, proteins and fibre-rich (unrefined) carbohydrates are still needed. In the following pages we teach you how to turn macronutrient advice (fat, proteins and carbohydrates) into real foods and patterns of eating. Don't forget: all fats, whether they are saturated or unsaturated, are high in calories. This calorie load is the same whether the fat is solid at room temperature (as in butter), or liquid (as in vegetable oils). It is therefore important for our health and our waistlines that we watch the amount of fat and fatty foods we eat. The main messages from these pages are set out in the table at the end of this section.

Monounsaturated fats

Foods rich in monounsaturated fats include:

- Olive oil, rapeseed oil and spreads based on these
- Avocado
- Nuts, flaxseed, nut oils

Polyunsaturated fats

Foods rich in polyunsaturated fats include:

- Corn, safflower and sunflower oil and spreads based on these
- Oily fish such as salmon, trout, herring and mackerel
- Sunflower and other edible seeds

The main plant-based oils that we eat in the UK are sunflower, rapeseed, olive, corn and soybean oils. They each contain a unique blend of unsaturated and saturated fatty acids.

Fatty acid composition of culinary oils
(Foster R, Williamson CS, and Lunn J 2009)

	Total fat g/100 g	Saturates g/100 g	Monounsaturates g/100 g	Polyunsaturates g/100 g
Sunflower oil	99.9	12.0	20.5	63.3
Rapeseed oil	99.9	6.6	59.3	29.3
Corn oil	99.9	14.4	29.9	51.3
Soybean oil	99.9	15.6	21.3	58.8
Olive oil	99.9	14.3	73.0	8.2
Flaxseed oil	99.9	9.4	20.2	66.0
Peanut oil	99.9	20.0	44.4	31.0
Walnut oil	99.9	9.1	16.5	69.9
Sesame oil	99.7	14.6	37.5	43.4
Safflower oil	99.9	9.7	12.0	74.0

What are omega-3, −6 and −9 fatty acids?

Omega-3, omega-6 and omega-9 fatty acids are all unsaturated fats, so they all have double bonds within their structure. The number just refers to the position of the first double bond. So omega-3s have their first double bond on carbon number 3 (counting from the methyl end of the carbon chain) and so on.

All unsaturated fats (omega-3, −6 or −9) have a role in promoting good health so it's good to get a balance between all three.

Scientists tend to refer to these different fats as families. Each family has a parent fatty acid. In the case of the omega-3 fatty acid family, the parent is alpha linolenic acid (usually abbreviated to ALA). It is one of the two essential fats. The other essential fat is linoleic acid (LA) and this is the parent omega-6 fatty acid. Both of these fats have an 18-carbon backbone. We have to eat foods that contain both linoleic and alpha linolenic acid because we cannot make them ourselves. While it is usually easy to source omega-6 and −9 fats from vegetable and seed oils, omega-3s are less plentiful in the typical British diet.

In theory, we can make more omega-3 and −6 fatty acids from these two parents just by adding on more carbon atoms. In practice it is not so easy. There is good evidence that the rate of conversion of the essential omega-3 fatty acid − ALA − to the longer chain fatty acids EPA and DHA is very slow, particularly so in men. As these fats have some very potent anti-inflammatory effects in the body, a dietary source is very wise. Our UK dietary guidelines advise an intake of 450 mgs of EPA and DHA combined per day, or around 3–3.5 g per week. This can be achieved through one good portion of oily fish per week.

Main omega-3 fatty acids

Types of omega-3 fatty acids	Main sources
ALA – alpha-linolenic acid	Rapeseed, soybeans, walnut and oils made from these dark green vegetables
EPA – eicosapentaenoic acid	Oily fish such as kippers, fresh tuna, mackerel, pilchards, trout. Also produced from algae
DHA – docosahexaenoic acid	

What counts as oily fish?

Oily fish (provides on average 2 g of EPA and DHA per 100 g)	White fish (provides on average 0.3 g of EPA and DHA per 100 g	Shellfish (provides on average 0.4 g of EPA and DHA per 100 g)
Mackerel	Cod	Prawns
Kipper	Plaice	Crabs
*Tuna (fresh/frozen)	Haddock	Lobsters
Salmon	Coley	Mussels
Herring	Whiting	Cockles
Pilchards	Skate	Oysters
Sardines	Red Snapper	Scallops
Swordfish	Sea bream	Clams
Whitebait	Turbot	
Kipper	Marlin	
Anchovies	Tinned tuna	
Eel	Sea bass	
Bloater	Red and grey mullet	
Carp	Halibut	
Sprats	Lemon and Dover sole	
	Parrot fish	
	Shark	
	Hake	

*Fresh tuna is rich in omega-3 fats, but when it's canned these fats are reduced to levels similar to white fish. This means that only fresh tuna can be regarded as an oil-rich fish.

If choosing canned or smoked fish be aware that some varieties can be high in salt. Try to choose fish that has been sustainably caught or farmed. You can check this information on the packaging or online.

White fish and shellfish are particularly low in fat, making them a great choice if you are trying to cut down your total fat intake, but try to have a mix of fish types each week. Unfortunately some deep-sea and oily fish (swordfish, marlin, shark) contain trace amounts of natural pollutants so we need to ensure we don't over-consume these foods. The following advice has been issued by the Department of Health following a review of the composition and possible health effects.

Best practice advice

	Men and boys and women not intending to become pregnant	Women of childbearing age, pregnant and breastfeeding women
General advice	At least 2 portions* of fish per week, 1 of which should be oily	At least 2 portions of fish per week, 1 of which should be oily. No more than two portions a week of • dogfish (rock salmon) • sea bass • sea bream • turbot • halibut • crab
Caution	No more than 4 portions of oily fish per week. Up to one portion of swordfish, marlin or shark per week	No more than 2 portions of oily fish per week. No more than two tuna steaks per week or 4 cans of tuna Avoid swordfish, marlin and shark Breastfeeding women do not need to limit tuna intake but should have no more than one portion of swordfish, marlin or shark per week)

*one portion = 140 g/5oz

The heart-protective effects of ALA, EPA and DHA

Interest in the heart-protective effects of omega-3 fatty acids (ALA, EPA, DHA) began with the observation that the Inuit people of Greenland rarely died from coronary heart disease, despite their high-fat diet largely derived from seafood.

Good evidence has shown that a regular intake of omega-3 fatty acids can reduce the number of sudden fatal heart attacks in people at high risk of cardiovascular disease. More recent research has raised some doubts, but the likely explanation why these recent trials showed no benefit is that the studies recruited too few people to show a beneficial effect. In addition, any positive effect that we expected to see might have been masked by the far more potent medications (such as cholesterol and blood-pressure lowering drugs) which the subjects were taking in these studies and which were not available to those individuals in the original studies.

Despite these more recent studies health professionals, dietitians and lipid experts still believe omega-3 fatty acids from oily fish have a crucial role to play in a heart-healthy diet. Their effects include:

- Reducing the stickiness of blood, so that it's less likely to clot
- Helping to keep the heart beating regularly
- Protecting the small arteries that carry blood to the heart from damage
- Lowering the amount of triglycerides in the blood
- Reducing blood pressure.

The amount required to gain these benefits varies but an intake of around 450 mg to 1 g of EPA plus DHA each day is a good starting point. This can be achieved by including one to two portions of oily fish per week.

Improving the balance of saturated to unsaturated fats

Reduce saturated and trans fats:	By reducing animal fats: • Butter, ghee, lard, dripping, suet, hard margarines and foods made from these (cakes, biscuits, puddings, pies, pastries and pasties) • Dairy produce (full-cream milk, cheese, full-fat yoghurt, crème fraîche and cream) • Fatty meats and meat products (sausages, burgers, salami) By reducing some key vegetable fats: • Palm and coconut oils By reducing processed foods; especially: • Foods labelled with partially hydrogenated vegetable fat/oil or high in saturated fat • Takeaways

Replace saturated fat and trans fats with unsaturated fats	By using: • Nut, olive and seed oils in cooking and salad dressings • Swapping butter for unsaturated spreads and lard for vegetable oil • Incorporating unsalted nuts and seeds, avocado into more meals and snacks • Cooking more from basic ingredients • Choose oily fish at least once a week
Practical ways to increase omega-3 intake from vegetable sources (AHA): • Choose rapeseed, soya, walnut, linseed (flaxseed) oils for food preparation and salad dressings • Eat walnuts as a snack or add to a salad • Sprinkle ground linseeds (flaxseeds) over porridge cereals, soups and salads. You can buy linseeds in most large supermarkets and health food stores • Eat a variety of dark green vegetables and green salad leaves • Eat more soya-based dishes such as tofu, soya beans, soya mince (see pages 197–248 for recipes)	
Practical ways to increase EPA and DHA: • Eat fish at least twice per week, one of which should be oily • Buy fresh fish in season and look out for special offers at the local supermarket and the fishmonger • Canned fish is convenient and cheap; frozen fish can be as nutritious as fresh • Serve canned fish on toast, in sandwiches or in jacket potatoes • Enjoy a posh brunch at the weekend by adding smoked salmon to scrambled eggs • Make tinned sardines into a pâté by mixing them with fromage frais, lemon zest and herbs • Make your own fish fingers, fish cakes or goujons with fresh salmon • If you or your family aren't too keen on fish, try making a fish pie to get used to the taste and texture	

Omega-6 fatty acids

Omega-6 fatty acids are also a kind of polyunsaturated fat. Linoleic acid, the parent omega-6 fatty acid, is essential for human health because it cannot be made in the body. Sources of omega-6 fatty acids include soybean oil, corn oil, safflower oil, peanut oil, sunflower oil, meat, egg yolks and vegetable spreads.

Our diet generally provides an abundant omega-6 intake (from oils and spreads), but is inadequate in omega-3 fats due to their being present in relatively few foods. A healthy diet should consist of roughly two to four times more omega-6 fatty acids than omega-3 fatty acids. However a typical diet may contain 11 to 20 times more omega-6 fatty acids than omega-3 fatty acids, and it is thought that this may promote inflammation and contribute to the development of diseases such as coronary heart disease and arthritis.

Omega-9 fatty acids

Omega-9 fatty acids are a family of unsaturated fats that are commonly found in vegetable and animal foods. Unlike omega-3 and omega-6 fatty acids, there are no essential omega-9 fatty acids as they can all be produced by the body, but they are also beneficial when they are obtained in food. Sources include rapeseed oil, sunflower oil, nut oils and almonds.

Summary

- Most foods contain some fat. The fat in food is usually a mixture of unsaturated and saturated fats.
  - Vegetables, cereals, nuts, seeds, soya and fish contain more unsaturated fats than saturated fat.
  - Animal products (meat, dairy foods), coconut and palm oils contain more saturated fat than unsaturated fat.
  - Harmful trans fats come from industrial processing and from heating unsaturated fats to high temperatures.
- While a heart-healthy diet is not a low-fat diet, take care with spreading fats, oil-based salad dressings and cooking oils as these are high in calories. Use them in small amounts.
- For your heart health it is important to replace saturated and trans fats with modest amounts of unsaturated (monounsaturated and polyunsaturated) fats.
- All kinds of unsaturated fats (whether they are omega-3, –6 or –9) have a role in promoting good health but it is important to get a balance between all three.

Stage 2: Cholesterol-busting foods

Adopting the cardio-protective diet we have described in the earlier part of this chapter will help to lower your cholesterol.

How much will depend upon how big a change you are able to make. Some people reading this book will already have a fairly healthy diet and others may be eating very poorly. The scope you have to make a difference to your cholesterol levels by adopting the Mediterranean style of eating will be different. At the very least you can expect to lower your cholesterol by 5 per cent, but this may be as high as 10 per cent or even 15 per cent if you make radical changes to a very poor diet.

Most of the changes made so far have focused on eating a varied diet with plenty of fruit, vegetables and wholegrains. We have encouraged you to identify the main sources of saturated fat in your diet and to reduce and replace these with healthy fats, such as those found in oily fish, seeds and nuts, and oils and spreads made from these.

Before you progress to the next stage it is important that you ensure that the foundations of your new cardio-protective diet are fully established. Forging healthy habits takes patience, time and effort. It is easy to slip back into the old patterns of eating if you are not careful so give yourself some time to adapt.

Once you are confident that your new diet is well established and you are comfortable with your new style of eating it's time to progress. But you should only do this if you are ready and when you consider it a priority for you now. If something else more pressing is taking much of your energy then it may be best to leave this next stage for a few weeks until you are able to focus all your resources on it. It might help you to revisit the chapter on motivation to help you make the decision as to when the time is right for you.

The portfolio diet

The portfolio diet describes a particular pattern of eating made popular by David Jenkins, a clinical researcher in Toronto, Canada. Professor Jenkins was well aware that certain foods have the potential to lower cholesterol levels by small but significant amounts when taken in sufficient quantities. He decided to test a theory. He believed that if four cholesterol-lowering foods were added together in a single eating plan (which he named the portfolio diet) then the total cholesterol-lowering effect of each ingredient might be additive.

His initial research was on a fairly small scale, using about 50 people with high cholesterol who attended his outpatient clinic and followed a test diet for a month. Each person was assigned to one of three groups:

a) The standard cholesterol-lowering diet (low in saturated fat and rich in wholegrains)
b) A low-intensity statin plus the standard cholesterol-lowering diet
c) The experimental portfolio diet.

The results were impressive. Those following the standard cholesterol-lowering diet had average LDL-cholesterol reductions of 8 per cent while the patients on the statin and standard diet lowered their LDL cholesterol by an average of 30 per cent. The patients on the new portfolio diet (but no statin) managed to lower their cholesterol by as much as 28 per cent on average, almost as much as those receiving the standard diet and statin therapy.

Three years after publishing this initial work, Jenkins went on to investigate if the same portfolio diet could be sustained over a longer 12–month period. He wanted to determine if this approach might deliver the same impressive results but over the longer term.

The average LDL-cholesterol-lowering effect was around 13 per cent. But Jenkins showed that about a third of the individuals were able to lower their cholesterol by more than 20 per cent. He also showed that higher levels of cholesterol lowering were obtained by those motivated individuals who stuck more rigidly to the key elements of the portfolio approach. However, even those people who were less dietary compliant, and ate less of the four portfolio foods than was prescribed, still made significant reductions above what would have been expected from the standard dietary approach.

Because of this research the four key elements of the portfolio diet have gained widespread recognition among diet experts as cholesterol-busting foods. However, the portfolio approach still appears to be under-used, perhaps because doctors and nurses are still unaware of its benefits or because few dietary resources are available to promote it. Without the appropriate resources, such as diet sheets, recipes and teaching aids, health professionals find it difficult to advise and support their patients appropriately.

The Ultimate Cholesterol-lowering Plan (UCLP©)

The Ultimate Cholesterol-Lowering Plan, or UCLP for short, is the UK's response to the portfolio diet. Brought up to date for a UK audience by HEART UK – The Cholesterol Charity – and based upon more recent knowledge, the UCLP is a step-by-step approach to cholesterol-lowering. The UCLP forms the second stage of our dietary journey to lower your cholesterol level.

So having described the background to the UCLP, it is time to introduce the cholesterol-busting foods. We recommend you read the remainder of this chapter before deciding on your own approach. We suggest that you tackle each food one at a time, as it may make things simpler for you. Start with the food type you think will be the easiest to introduce and establish a place for it in your eating plan. Don't think about moving on to the next food until you are ready to make that change. Adopting each food may take you as little as two weeks or as much as two months. Remember to take it at your own pace.

Cholesterol-busting food no. 1: nuts

Jenkins' portfolio diet used almonds, but all tree nuts have a similar nutritional profile so we recommend using a variety of nuts to meet this element of the diet. Tree nuts include almonds, Brazil nuts, cashews, hazelnuts, macadamia nuts, pecans, pine nuts and walnuts. Not only are they all rich in monounsaturated fats, plant proteins and fibre; they also contain good quantities of the essential fats and micronutrients such as vitamin E, folic acid, niacin, vitamin B_6, potassium, magnesium, copper, selenium, and naturally occurring phytonutrients such as sterols and phenolic antioxidants.

Nuts are both high in calories and fat. This is perhaps why doctors and other health professionals have been reluctant to recommend or endorse them to their patients. When encouraging people to eat nuts one of the most common responses we get is 'I thought eating nuts would make me gain weight, which is bad for my heart. The doctor told me to avoid them!'

It is true, nuts are high in calories, and although most of the fat found in nuts is unsaturated, most nuts cannot be described as low in saturated fat either. However, studies have consistently shown that regular nut consumption does not result in weight gain. While we are not entirely sure why this is, it could be for two reasons. Firstly, nuts are high in fat, protein and vegetable fibre, which together appear to have an effect in suppressing our appetite. So, eating nuts regularly appears to help you feel fuller for longer. The second reason is that the energy contained in nuts is unlikely to be fully available to the body. We just can't access it. Why? Because all of the energy is tightly packaged up inside the cells of nuts. When we eat nuts we only break them into small pieces by chewing, releasing only a fraction of the nut oil. Further digestion lower in the gut seems unable to access much of the remaining oil.

Chestnuts, also a tree nut, are very different to others in the family. They contain only very small amounts of fat, so it is debatable if they deliver the cardio-protective benefits of other tree nuts.

Despite their name, peanuts or ground nuts are not a nut, in fact they are a legume. However their nutritional profile is sufficiently similar to those of other nuts so we include them in the options for your regular nut intake.

Coconut is the exception. Almost all (85 per cent) of the fat in coconut is saturated. The main saturated fatty acid in coconut is lauric acid. It has been suggested that lauric acid has beneficial properties because it increases HDL cholesterol more than other saturated fatty acids. However, lauric acid also increases total and LDL cholesterol more than other fatty acids, making it the most atherogenic of all the fatty acids. Research is still going on about the health benefits (or otherwise) of coconut oil, so until results are more conclusive it is best to avoid coconut oil and creamed coconut, and to use coconut milk sparingly too.

The easiest way to include nuts regularly in your diet is as a snack, but they can be included in recipes too, either as a complete replacement for the animal protein or as an accompaniment.

Cholesterol-busting food no. 2: soya foods

The humble soya bean is a legume which is packed full of nutrients and is becoming increasingly popular in westernised diets. Soya is about 40 per cent protein, 20 per cent fat and 20 per cent fibre, the remainder being water and a small amount of carbohydrate. The protein in soya is what we call 'high biological value', meaning it is of good quality and can sustain both growth and repair of human tissues. For this reason it can be used to replace animal proteins in the diet without causing any adverse effects on either growth or development. The fat in the soya bean is mainly unsaturated. Soya beans are also rich in calcium and magnesium.

Soya has come in for some criticism over recent years. This is because of certain substances in soya which are similar in structure to the female hormone oestrogen. However their effects are much, much weaker. Collectively these are known as phytoestrogens, but are often referred to as soya isoflavones. They have been shown to have both oestrogenic and anti-oestrogenic actions. Some concerns have arisen that these phytoestrogens may have unwanted health effects in humans such as increasing the risk of breast and prostate cancer, or causing an underactive thyroid. It has also been suggested that phytoestrogens might be beneficial in preventing or reducing some of the effects of the menopause such as hot flushes and bone loss. Epidemiological studies of populations that eat diets rich in soy over many, many years have not shown any increase in cancers and in fact people who eat a traditional Chinese and Japanese diet usually have lower levels of heart disease, cancers and menopausal symptoms. Scientists have evaluated the findings from laboratory, animal and human studies and as a result have concluded that regular soya intake has no detrimental effect, and in fact has the potential to reduce breast cancer risk.

Evidence shows that incidence of breast cancer is actually lowest in high soy-eating communities such as Asia and highest in Western communities. There appears to be a modest reduction in risk from breast cancer when soy intake is increased. Furthermore, this effect seems to be greater the more soy that is eaten and when intake starts early in childhood.

Further concerns, from people with existing breast or prostate cancer, that soy consumption might exacerbate their condition are also unfounded. Soy foods, even at the higher intake levels, appear to have no negative influence on the recurrence of either breast or prostate cancer and may in some cases significantly reduce the risk.

So that sounds like good news. Soy foods fall into two categories, fermented and non-fermented soya foods:

Fermented soya foods include tempeh (a firm soya cake widely used in Indonesia), natto (a sticky, slimy soy fermented product that is often used as a breakfast food in Japan) and miso (a thick paste usually used for flavouring soups, sauces and for spreading in Japanese cooking). Soya sauce is also a fermented product and common ingredient used in Asian cooking. It is very salty, low in fat and contains about 10 g protein per 100 ml. Given its use as a condiment in smallish quantities it provides little nutritional benefit to the diet but can significantly increase the salt content of Asian dishes.

Non-fermented soya foods are perhaps the most familiar to us as they tend to be used more in Western diets. These include immature soya beans (edamame beans); which can be used as a simple vegetable or in salads; the roasted soya bean, which is often referred to as soya nuts; and tofu (a curd made from soya beans). Soya milk, soya desserts and yoghurt alternatives are also growing in popularity in the UK. Many processed foods now contain soy, and soya mince and soya chunks are available in many health food stores.

Soya foods appear to have two main ways of lowering LDL cholesterol. Just by replacing animal proteins (like meat and cheese) with soya proteins, we significantly reduce our saturated fat intake and increase our consumption of the more healthy unsaturated fats. The second effect is caused by a change in cholesterol metabolism inside the body. The nature of this is not entirely known but the likely explanation is that soy protein may inhibit cholesterol synthesis in the liver and so reduce overall LDL-cholesterol levels.

Cholesterol-busting food no. 3: soluble fibre

Plant fibres come in two distinct forms: insoluble and soluble. Neither form of fibre has any calorific value and both are important to the body because of the vital role they play in keeping our gut healthy. They help:

- Speed up the rate of digestion
- Prevent constipation and other gut disorders such as hiatus hernia, diverticulitis, haemorrhoids and bowel cancer
- Maintain a healthy balance of good bacteria in the lower bowel.

   Soluble fibre has been shown to have cholesterol-lowering properties. It dissolves in water in the gut to form a gel-like substance, which can only be described as similar to wallpaper paste! But instead of sticking to the walls of your intestines, it soaks up cholesterol, like a sponge, and carries it out of the body where it cannot do any damage.

Soluble fibre is found in varying quantities in many cereals, pulses, fruits and vegetables. Oats, oat bran and barley contain a special form of soluble fibre called beta glucan. This is one of the most effective forms of soluble fibre.

Cholesterol-busting food no. 4: plant sterol and stanol-fortified foods and supplements

Plant sterols and stanols are naturally present in very small quantities in many plant foods including wholegrains, plant oils, vegetables and nuts. Most of us in the UK have intakes of around 300 mg per day. Plant stanols and sterols are the vegetable kingdom's equivalent of cholesterol. They have a chemical structure which is very similar to cholesterol and when consumed at high enough doses, they compete with cholesterol in the gut for absorption. This reduces cholesterol absorption and increases its elimination via faeces. So just like soluble fibre, plant sterols and stanols affect the absorption of cholesterol but in a slightly different way. The effect is the same though: both lower LDL cholesterol by preventing the recycling of cholesterol and bile acids.

The amount of plant sterols and stanols needed to achieve any significant effect is more than we can get from a normal diet. Hence a whole industry has grown up over recent years providing a range of plant sterol and stanol-fortified foods and supplements.

Both sterols and stanols work in the same way and have equivalent effects. Foods that have been fortified with plant sterols and stanols are well researched and over 200 clinical trials have shown conclusively that they lower cholesterol very effectively. Food supplements containing plant sterols have been less well researched. It is possible that they may not work as well but no one knows for sure. Look out for a range of fortified foods such as spreads, yoghurts, milks, shots and cheeses in the chilled supermarket aisles. There are two main brands of fortified foods in the UK – Benecol and Flora Pro.Activ – but many retailers have developed own-label versions. Foods fortified with plant sterols and stanols are the only one of our super foods that **cannot** be eaten universally by everyone. This is because they have a slightly greater cholesterol-lowering effect than nuts, soy foods or soluble fibre and because they can affect the absorption of other nutrients. Here are the key recommendations to bear in mind when taking these products:

- You need to ensure you take enough stanol/sterol-fortified products to achieve the effective dose
- Don't consume more than the effective dose as this is unlikely to result in greater cholesterol-lowering
- Stanol/sterol-fortified products should only be taken with meals to optimise their impact
- They should not be taken by pregnant or breastfeeding women, children and those with normal cholesterol levels
- These products may have a small effect on the absorption of fat-soluble vitamins. To compensate, ensure you eat plenty of fruit and vegetables.

Putting the science into practice – how much to eat

Nuts

Cholesterol-lowering effect: 3–5%
How much: 30–35 g per day
Eaten as: a snack or as part of a meal

What does 30 g of nuts look like?

Nut	Number to make 30 g		
Almonds	20	Peanuts	30
Brazil nuts	10	Pecans	15
Cashews	15	Pine nuts	2 tablespoons
Hazelnuts	21	Walnuts	10
Macadamia nuts	15		

As a rule of thumb, for every 10 g of nuts you eat, you can expect to lower your LDL cholesterol by 1 per cent.

Soya foods

Cholesterol-lowering effect: 4–5%
How much: aim for 15 g of soy protein per day – that's 1–3 portions of soya foods per day dependent upon which you choose
Eaten as: snack (soya nuts), dessert, replacement for cows' milk (soya milk), as a meat replacement, as a vegetable or part of a salad (edamame beans).

Common soya foods and their protein content

Food	Amount of protein	Food	Amount of protein
Soya nuts (28 g)	15 g	Tofu (100 g)	Range 7–18 g
Cooked mature soya beans (85 g)	14 g	Miso (25 g)	3 g
Edamame beans (80 g)	8.5 g		
Soya burger (75 g)	10 g		
Soya milk (250 ml)	7.5 g		
Soya yoghurt (150 g)	5–6g		
Soya dessert	5 g		
Soya texturised meat replacement (25 g dry weight)	12 g		

Soluble fibre

Cholesterol-lowering effect: 5%
How much: aim for 2–3 portions of oats and barley each day to provide 3 g beta glucan
Eaten as: **oats** – porridge or an oat-based breakfast cereal, as oat bran sprinkled on cereal, in smoothies, soups, casseroles, oatcakes, fish coated with oats, oats in bread and other low-saturated fat recipes
barley – in soups and casseroles or as a replacement for rice.

Other soluble-fibre foods

Pulses: try to include one bean, pea or lentil portion per day
Fruits and vegetables: at least five a day (particularly okra, aubergine and pectin-rich fruits such as citrus fruits, strawberries, apples).

Soluble fibre – how to achieve 3 g of beta glucan daily

Choose **three** from the list below:

- A bowl of porridge (using 30 g of porridge oats)
- 2 tablespoons of oat bran – sprinkled on to cereals or added to casseroles, soups or smoothies
- 1 oat breakfast biscuit
- 1 serving of oat bran cereal
- 3 oatcakes
- 30 g of oats in recipes that are also low in saturated fat
- 2 slices or 1 roll of bread with a high percentage of oat content (check labels)
- 150 g cooked pearl barley – added to stews, casseroles, in salads or use instead of rice to make a risotto
- 40 g serving of barley flakes.

Plant sterols and stanols

Cholesterol-lowering effect: 7–10%
How much: 1.5–2.4 g per day
Eat as: **either** 1 mini fortified yoghurt shot per day (providing around 2 g) **or** 2–3 portions of a fortified spread, yoghurt or milk per day (each portion provides around 0.75 g)

NB A portion is 2 teaspoons of fortified spread, 200 ml glass of fortified milk, 1 fortified yoghurt

Sample menu

Breakfast: Oatmeal porridge made with 150 ml soya milk topped with chopped almonds
Lunch: Jacket potato with baked beans and salad served with an oat and fruit smoothie
Evening meal: Salmon steak coated in oats and pan fried in a little sunflower oil served with new potatoes, okra and carrots. Plant sterol or stanol yoghurt shot
Snacks/drinks: One serving of fruit and a handful of soya nuts or roasted Edamame beans.

For more meal ideas check out the recipes at the back of this book or visit the HEART UK website www.heartuk.org.uk/UCLP

Summary

- Cholesterol-busting foods can play an active part in helping to lower your cholesterol
  - Nuts
  - Soya and other vegetable proteins
  - Soluble fibre (from oats, barley, pulses, fruits and vegetables)
  - Plant sterol and stanol-fortified foods
- The cholesterol-lowering effect of these foods is modest but it is also additive – the more you have the bigger the effect
- It's best to start with one of these foods and establish it as part of your dietary routine before progressing to the next.

Food labelling

Recent changes in food labelling mean that our labels are now clearer to understand and offer more information than ever before. You can check exactly what you are eating from the nutritional breakdown; any key ingredients you would prefer not to consume (such as allergens or partially hydrogenated fats); the best before or use by date; the specific country the food originates from; and any special storage, cooking or warning information.

The introduction of food-labelling information on the front of pre-packaged foods is a really helpful tool. Not only is it designed to help keep you informed about what you are buying; it can also assist you in making healthier choices because you are able to see the energy, fat, sugar and salt content of a food at a glance. Retailer research shows that more people are using this front-of-pack information to compare one product against a similar product before they decide to purchase.

Nutrition and health claims

The claims that foods can make on their packs, in advertising and promotional materials are highly regulated across Europe. There are two main kinds of claims that foods can make.

- **Nutrition claim** – such as reduced fat, low salt, no added sugars, high in fibre
- **Health claim** – such as:
  - Calcium and vitamin D are needed for normal growth and development of bones
  - Vitamin C increases iron absorption
  - Plant sterols and plant stanol esters have been shown to lower/reduce blood cholesterol; high cholesterol is a risk factor in the development of coronary heart disease
  - Beta glucans contribute to the maintenance of normal blood cholesterol levels.

The fact that nutrition and health claims are so highly regulated is good for the consumer. It provides peace of mind and reassurance, which together enable the general public to trust our food labels. If a claim is not made on a product it's likely that there is a good reason for it. Either the nutrition or health claim has not been approved by the regulatory body, or the food does not qualify under the conditions of use.

Look out for products that carry cholesterol-lowering claims

Foods that contain 1 g or more of beta glucans, in a recognised single portion, from either oats or barley

> What the claim might look like: *Oat/barley beta glucan has been shown to lower/reduce blood cholesterol. High cholesterol is a risk factor in the development of coronary heart disease.*

Foods low in saturated fat and/or rich in unsaturated fats

> What the claim might look like: *Replacing saturated fats with unsaturated fats in the diet has been shown to lower/reduce blood cholesterol. High cholesterol is a risk factor in the development of coronary heart disease.*

Foods fortified with plant sterol and plant stanol esters

> What the claim might look like: *Plant sterols/stanols have been shown to lower/reduce blood cholesterol. High cholesterol is a risk factor in the development of coronary heart disease. The beneficial effect can be obtained with a daily intake of 1.5–2.4 g plant sterols/stanols over 2–3 weeks.*

The European Food Safety Authority (EFSA) maintains a register of all authorised nutrition and health claims and their conditions for use, and these can be accessed online at: http://ec.europa.eu/nuhclaims/

Reference Intakes

From December 2014 all new food packs should use the term Reference Intake (RI). The RI is the amount of a nutrient needed every day to ensure that most people receive an adequate amount to cover their individual needs.

For simplicity there is only one set of figures to cover all groups of the population. The RI is mainly aimed at adults and is based on an average woman with energy needs of around 2,000 kilocalories (8400 kilojoules) per day. These figures have been agreed by the European Food Safety Authority for labelling purposes. It is important to note that the RI's for fat, saturates, sugar and salt are all maximums and not targets to be aimed for.

Ingredients list

All the ingredients in a food are listed on the pack in descending order by weight. So the first ingredient in the list will be present in the greatest quantity. The amount of a specific ingredient may have to be stated if it is mentioned in the food name or if it is emphasised on the label in words or by pictures (e.g., picture of a strawberry on a strawberry yoghurt, or beef and potato in a beef and potato pie).

Oils and fats may be grouped together on an ingredient list, for example, as 'vegetable oils' but the source of the oils will have to follow this (e.g., palm, coconut, sunflower, rapeseed) with the oil present in the largest amount coming first.

Industrially hydrogenated oils (a potential source of harmful trans fats) have to be labelled within the ingredient list as either fully hydrogenated fats or partially hydrogenated fats. Only partially hydrogenated fats are a source of harmful trans fats and ideally should be avoided. Fully hydrogenated fats are saturated fats and should be limited.

The ingredient list is also very helpful if you want to look for and avoid specific ingredients, such as a food or ingredient you might be allergic to.

Front-of-pack labelling

Most packaged foods and drink products show simple nutritional information on the front of their packs. This is a voluntary scheme in the UK. This label is usually prominent on the front of the pack and shows the energy content of the foods and in most cases the fat, saturates, sugars and salt it contains. Information is provided per portion, for example, half a pizza, or two sausages. It gives instant information both about the normal portion size and what it contains.

The scheme also allows for traffic-light colour-coding to indicate whether a nutrient such as saturates is present in high (red) medium (amber) or low (green) amounts. In reality, only a few foods will qualify as green on all four criteria (fat, saturates, sugar and salt). So, as a guide, for a food to qualify as a healthy choice on your menu look for:

- The best in the category when compared against similar products
- A mixture of greens and ambers and very few reds
- Where the food contributes other essential nutrients to the diet e.g. iron, calcium, protein, vitamins and minerals.

You can use front-of-pack labelling information in many ways including:

a) To check on specific nutrients that you are interested in – e.g., saturated fat
b) To choose between two similar foods
c) To choose a food that best meets your needs
d) To understand how much a portion contributes to your nutrient intake
e) To see how individual foods can fit into a healthy balanced diet.

A word about drinks

The low-, medium- and high-nutrient boundaries for drinks are half of those for foods. You can use these in exactly the same way as you use the criteria for foods.

Drinks that contain sugars that come from crushed fruit, fruit juice or from milk are considered to be healthier than drinks containing added sugars. This is simply because milk, juices and smoothies contribute other nutrients to the diet and contain fewer artificial ingredients. Take care with flavoured milk and milk-based drinks as these may contain a little more added sugar.

Drinks are very easy to consume and pass through our stomachs relatively quickly so generally they don't satisfy our appetites in the same way as foods. They can also contain a lot of calories in the form of fat, sugar or alcohol and often few other nutrients.

Summary

- Checking the nutrition information on food labels will help you to make sure you and your family are eating a healthy balanced diet
- Look out for front-of-pack labelling on all kinds of pre-prepared foods
- Use it to compare two or more foods from the same category against each other
- Be aware of the health claims on food packs – if the product does not make a claim, chances are it can't
- Become familiar with the way foods display the nutrition information on packs
- Look out for sources of unwanted saturated fat (e.g., hydrogenated fat, palm oil, coconut oil, lard, butter, dairy fat, meat fat, cream) especially if high up the ingredient list; you can check the total saturated fat per 100 g in the saturated fat declaration in the nutrition information panel

- Look out for sources of unwanted trans fats (partially hydrogenated fat/oil) in the list of ingredients on food packaging.

Dietary swaps

You can help keep your heart healthy by swapping a few items in your diet. This guide is not meant to be exhaustive. We encourage you to read food labels (see pages 133–7) to find out just how much saturated fat is in specific products before you decide to buy.

Food swaps

Dairy products	
Swap this	**For this**
Full-fat milk	1 per cent fat or skimmed milk
Evaporated milk	Evaporated fat-free or reduced-fat milk
Double cream	Low-fat yoghurt
Cream	Reduced-fat crème fraîche or yoghurt; soya or oat cream alternatives
Sour cream	Plain low-fat yoghurt
Hard cheese (e.g. Cheddar)	Cottage cheese or reduced-fat cheese
Creamy or cheese sauces for meat/pasta	Tomato or vegetable-based sauces
Butter	Sunflower, olive, soya, sterol/stanol spreads
Ice cream, especially dairy	Sorbet, low-fat ice cream or fat-free frozen yoghurt
Latte made with whole milk	Skinny latte
Full-fat dips	Low-fat yoghurt dips
Meat, poultry and fish	
Regular minced beef/lamb	Extra lean mince or chicken/turkey mince
Pork belly	Lean pork steaks
Streaky bacon	Grilled lean back bacon, rind removed
Steak-and-kidney pie	Cottage pie

Cured fatty meats, like salami	Ham, chicken or turkey slices
Fried sausages	Grilled low-fat meat or vegetarian sausages
Chicken thigh with skin on	Chicken breast with skin removed
Fried battered fish, especially if cooked in lard	Grilled or baked fish
Snacks	
Fried snacks (e.g. crisps)	Breadsticks, rice cakes or crunchy vegetables, air-popped popcorn
Cream cakes, pastries	Toasted currant buns, English muffins, crumpets, with a little unsaturated spread
Biscuits	Choose lowest in saturated fat
Bar of milk chocolate	Few pieces of dark chocolate
Miscellaneous	
Slice of pizza	Wholegrain pitta bread dipped in low-fat hummus or tzatziki
Chip-shop chips	Oven chips
Canned cream soups	Canned broth or tomato-based soups
Mayonnaise	Light or extra-light mayonnaise or mustard
Salad dressings	Olive oil or nut-oil-based dressings, reduced calorie or fat-free salad dressings

Meal ideas

To make life easier we have come up with a meal planner to help you with everyday heart-friendly meal and snack choices. You don't have to follow it to the letter, but it is meant to give you some ideas of the types of foods that you can fit into your new heart-healthy eating plan.

Here are some good tips for when you are planning meals:

- Make sure you include a variety of foods every day
- Try to include at least five portions of fruits and vegetables each day
- Build each meal around a starchy wholegrain food such as wholemeal bread, brown pasta or brown basmati rice
- Take care with your portion sizes

- Try to have three small meals a day rather than miss meals and then over indulge later
- Try to include foods from as many of the food groups as you can at each meal. The main food groups are:
  - Meat, fish, eggs and other non-dairy sources of protein such as nuts, lentils and soya alternatives to meat
  - Milk and dairy foods (choose low fat) or dairy alternatives such as soya milk
  - Fruit, vegetables, pulses
  - Bread, rice, potatoes, pasta and other starchy foods
- Try to include a variety of colours and textures on your plate
- Make a shopping list and stick to it.

Breakfast

Make time for breakfast. People who eat breakfast in the morning are less likely to be overweight.

Lunch

Since most of us tend to eat lunch outside the home, it can be problematic, limited by time, budget and availability. If you are a sandwich eater, and make your own, the variations are endless…

Tips for healthier sandwiches:

- Always use wholegrain varieties of bread
- Include 2–3 salad items such as tomato, cucumber, red or green bell pepper, onion or lettuce
- Use spreads high in unsaturated fats, mustard or light mayonnaise instead of butter or regular mayonnaise
- Choose from a wide range of sandwich fillers (e.g. canned salmon with cucumber; tuna with low-fat mayonnaise and celery; hummus and red pepper; banana and avocado; cooked lean meat or fish; cooked chicken with low-fat salad dressing and sweetcorn; boiled egg and low-fat mayonnaise; lean ham, mustard and watercress; peanut butter with sliced dates.

Dinner

Traditionally this is the main meal of the day – and the one where most of us overindulge! Plan what you are going to prepare ahead of time. It will pay off later when your energy and good intentions are flagging at the end of the day.

Water

Drink at least a glass of water with each of your three meals and with each snack.

Alcohol

Drink alcohol in moderation.

Sample meal planner

Menu Planner – Week 1

	Breakfast	Snack	Lunch	Snack	Evening meal
Monday	2 oatibix with soya milk and spiced puréed apple	Handful of mixed unsalted nuts	Lentil soup and granary roll	An apple	Salmon steak (To cook, cover the steak with chopped garlic, ginger and lemon juice and wrap in foil. Bake for 20 minutes.) Serve with new potatoes and large mixed salad. Sterol/stanol mini yoghurt drink
Tuesday	Spinach and mushroom 2-egg omelette with a slice of toasted soy and linseed bread with 2 tsp sterol/stanol-fortified spread	A handful of grapes	Sardines on wholegrain toast with 2 tsp sterol/stanol-fortified spread	2 oatcakes spread with peanut butter	Lean chicken stir fry with peppers, baby sweetcorn, green beans and broccoli florets. Serve with wholemeal tortillas, guacamole and tomato salsa
Wednesday	Porridge made with soya milk and topped with one tbsp dried fruit	A glass of carrot and orange juice	Jacket potato with sunflower spread, tuna, sweetcorn and light mayonnaise served with salad	Soya yoghurt alternative	Mexican bean tacos: fill warm tacos with mexi-beans and top with shredded lettuce, grated reduced-fat cheese and tomato salsa
Thursday	Home-made muesli (mixture of rolled oats, with dried fruit, nuts and seeds) with low-fat milk and a few sliced strawberries	A piece of fruit	Wholemeal pasta salad with corn, spring onion, red pepper, cherry tomatoes, olives and cucumber, and a little olive oil with sliced chicken strips. Sterol/stanol mini yoghurt drink	Handful of unsalted almonds	Spaghetti Bolognese using soya mince and canned red kidney beans instead of beef. Serve with wholegrain spaghetti and salad

	Breakfast	Snack	Lunch	Snack	Evening meal
Friday	Wholegrain toast spread with mashed avocado and topped with sliced fresh tomato and a little lemon juice	Fruit smoothie (To make blend low-fat milk, low-fat natural yoghurt, a banana and a handful of berries)	Chickpea salad: mix canned chickpeas, button mushrooms, diced red onion, red pepper with a little olive oil and vinaigrette dressing	Wholemeal hot-cross bun	Stir-fried lean beef with garlic, onion, red pepper, okra and mangetout dressed with sweet chilli sauce and served with brown rice
Saturday	Traditional rolled oats topped with fresh or frozen raspberries and soya yoghurt	Handful of soya nuts	Minestrone soup sprinkled with oat bran and served with a granary roll with 2 tsp sterol/stanol-fortified spread	A piece of fruit	Bake a firm white fish fillet in white wine (optional), lemon juice, chopped ginger, garlic and coriander for 20 minutes. Serve with a good helping of steamed vegetables and mashed sweet potato
Sunday	Baked beans and scrambled egg on soy and linseed toast	Handful of mixed unsalted nuts	Roast chicken. Serve with a generous helping of steamed vegetables and a few roast potatoes cooked in vegetable oil	Wholemeal English muffin spread with 2 tsp sterol/stanol-fortified spread	Soya burger served with baked beans and a large salad

Meal Planner Week 2

	Breakfast	Snack	Lunch	Snack	Evening meal
Monday	Oat fruit smoothie (Put a small banana, a handful of blueberries and 200 ml soya milk into a blender and mix until smooth. Stir in 2 tablespoons of fine oatmeal. Leave to chill in the fridge for an hour or so.)	Handful of mixed nuts and seeds	Mixed bean soup and wholegrain roll with 2 tsp sterol/stanol spread	2 oatcakes with hummus	Grilled lean lamb fillets with boiled sweet potatoes and broccoli
Tuesday	Poached egg with wilted spinach and grilled tomato with a slice of wholegrain bread with 1 tsp sterol/stanol-fortified spread	Handful of cherries or 1 apple	Fill a wholemeal pitta bread with mashed avocado, sliced cucumber and tomatoes, and shredded lettuce, dress with a little lemon juice	Small handful of dried fruit and nut mix	Tuna pasta with a tomato and cucumber salad
Wednesday	Chopped banana stirred into porridge made with low-fat milk, top with chopped almonds	Handful of dried apricots	3 bean mixed salad: mix canned 3 beans, diced red onion, red pepper and lemon juice	Hot chocolate made with low-fat milk	Grilled chicken breast with roasted sweet potatoes, and roasted Mediterranean vegetables
Thursday	Homemade muesli (see recipe)	A pear	Salmon and cucumber open sandwiches on rye bread	2 oatcakes with mashed avocado	Nut roast
Friday	Tomatoes and mushroom omelette with a slice of soya and linseed bread	Low-fat yoghurt	Jacket potato with tuna and sweetcorn and a large green salad	Fresh fruit	See recipe for prune and chicken tray bake
Saturday	Wholegrain toast with peanut butter	2 figs and 2 Brazil nuts	See recipe for Tuna Nicoise	Vegetable sticks and hummous	Chilli con carne made with lean beef mince and kidney beans, served with steamed brown rice and salad
Sunday	Mackerel on wholegrain toast with sliced tomatoes	Handful of soya nuts	See recipe for Cod with lime crushed new potatoes	Yoghurt with chopped-up grapes	Lentil bake

Keeping a food diary

Taking responsibility for your health is a huge part of making successful behavioural changes. Having someone to answer to, even if that person is yourself, is motivating and will keep you on track. A food diary is an important tool in developing dietary self-awareness, and one of the best ways to improve your eating habits. Recording everything you eat and drink gives you an accurate picture of what, when and why you eat. It's a good way to gain more control over your diet and lifestyle, since without recording what you eat, you might not notice dietary patterns, portion sizes, or the quality of your daily diet. Taking time to reflect on what and when you eat and drink before making any changes can help pinpoint simple changes you can easily make.

Recording what you eat, drink and how active you are can have several benefits:

Self-control

Just knowing that you have to write down everything you eat is a great deterrent. It might just give you that little extra self-control when it comes to saying no or overindulging in the wrong foods.

Identifying small changes

Keeping a food and drink diary, before you start to make changes, helps to establish your starting point. From here you can begin to explore the changes you are most comfortable making. Go for the easy ones first and establish them before moving on.

Identifying triggers

Keeping a detailed account of what, when and why you eat and drink can help you identify any important 'triggers' that prompt/precede particular eating or drink patterns. Just by recording what and when you eat, as well as your mood, you may start to notice patterns. For instance, are there types of food that you choose at certain stressful points in the day, or when you are dealing with particular emotions. Being aware of these habits can help you to confront and overcome them. Try thinking through different ways to avoid the 'trigger' completely or how you can modify your behaviour when faced by the same situation again.

Keeping track

A food diary is really helpful to look back on and can help you see what great progress you have made.

How to keep a food diary

- Your diary should be something that you are comfortable using on a regular basis without causing too much hassle. Ideally you should be able to record food on the go. Don't wait until the end of the day to record what you have eaten, chances are you will forget something important. You can write things down by hand, use a blank notebook or purchase a daily diary with enough space on each page to record your intake for the day (see page 148 for a sample diet diary page) or you can use an app or an online tracking device if you prefer.
- To start with, keep a diary for 7 days (including weekends) and then for at least 3 days a week on an ongoing basis. It's a good idea to include at least one day of the weekend as this is a time when you might eat or drink differently.
- Record everything you eat and drink in household measures, for example, 3 tablespoons of oats, half a glass of milk, 1 teaspoon sugar. Don't forget to record snacks and random odds and ends you eat, like a chocolate offered at work. Record your drinks as well, including your water intake. Try to be as detailed as you can. Be truthful!

- Make a note of where you ate, who you were with and how you were feeling at the time. This will help you figure out what life situations influence your eating.
- Consider recording your physical activities in the day, including day-to-day activities such as walking up a flight of steps at work, or 30 minutes washing the car, as well as more formal exercise, for example, a body pump class.

Analysing the data

- Use your diary to identify simple ways you could cut down on saturated fats or introduce healthy new foods. Make a note of two or three ideas and write these as SMART goals (see page 83).
- Look for patterns in your 7-day diary. When are you most vulnerable to eating or drinking the wrong things? Plan for these times. For example, save some cereal to have at 10 p.m. If you know evenings are a danger time, then make a list of ten other things you could do to distract yourself.
- Look for patterns in the triggers that cause you to eat unhealthily. Do you eat more when you're feeling angry, upset, lonely or bored? Is being home alone, watching TV, shopping when hungry, or having your meals prepared by someone else an issue? Noticing a pattern can help you plan how to make a change.
- Assess your snacking habits. Many people are surprised at how many snacks they actually eat in a given day. A biscuit with the mid-morning cup of tea, a chocolate bar in the car on the way back from work and munching on a bowl of crisps while watching TV at night can all add up. Use your diary to assess whether your snacking habits need an overhaul. If you tend to grab unhealthy snacks on the go, try thinking ahead and carry healthy snacks with you.
- Do you eat differently on non-work days? For most people, work has a big effect on their eating habits. If you work long hours you might find it hard to make time to cook properly. Do you tend to overindulge on alcohol at the weekend? Use this information to plan ahead.

Sample food and drink diary

What kind	How much	Time	Where	Alone or with whom	Activity	Mood
Coco-pops cereal with semi-skimmed milk	5 tbsp cereal & 1 glass milk	7.30 a.m.	Kitchen	Alone watching TV	Sitting	Tired
Chocolate biscuit	2	11 a.m.	Work	With colleague	Standing by the photo-copier	Bored
Can of Coke	1	12.30	Work	Alone	Sitting at desk	Happy
Ice-lolly	1	2 p.m.	Work	With colleague	Sitting at desk	Happy
Water	500 ml	5.30 p.m.	Gym	Alone	30 min on treadmill	happy
Pizza and salad	½ pizza, green salad, glass wine	7.30 p.m.	Home	With husband	Starving and needed something quick after the gym	In a rush to get out for the evening
2 glasses red wine and a packet of nuts	Large wine	9–10.30 p.m.	In the pub	With the girls – just winding down after a long day		Celebratory occasion – very happy
Doner kebab	Small pitta with 5 pieces of meat, salad and chilli sauce	11.15 p.m.	Kebab house	Still with the girls	Consensus decision to stop for something to eat on way home	Peckish, tipsy and tired

Eating out

Eating out is enjoyable. The occasional meal out won't make a difference to your cholesterol levels or health, so enjoy the treat. But if you are eating out regularly, say more than twice a week, this will have an impact on your overall food intake. Remember that an occasional café snack, takeaway pasty, 'quick bite' after work, and celebration meal all add up!

If your work or lifestyle dictate that you have to eat out a lot, it can be a challenge to stick to your preferred eating plan. But, with a little bit of pre-planning and using your knowledge to make healthy choices from the menu, it's still feasible.

Eating out tips

Before you go:

- Check what's on the menu. This will allow you to choose sensible options ahead of time. Recent changes mean that restaurants and fast-food chains now have to make the information about the ingredients in their recipes more available to customers on request. And in addition restaurants and fast-food chains are coming under more pressure to provide the calorie content of their food and drink on their menus and online. Having more information available makes it easier to decide what to eat before you even get to the restaurant.
- Take the edge off your hunger before you go out. Don't make the mistake of starving yourself all day only to overindulge when out.

At the restaurant:

- Take some plain bread from the bread basket, but avoid butter, garlic bread, or high-fat dips. Or better still ask the waiter to skip the bread basket. If you must have something to munch on while you wait for your order, ask for a plate of raw vegetables with a salsa dip or some breadsticks.

- Stick to only one or two courses. Consider a starter with a side order of vegetables instead of a main course or ask for a smaller portion.
- Don't be afraid to ask for your dishes to be adapted: vegetables without butter or sauces, or with the dressing on the side, plain salads as opposed to ones loaded with cheese, meat and salad dressings. Ask for lemon juice or oil-free dressing instead. If the item is fried, ask for it grilled.
- Go for dishes which are steamed, braised, grilled or baked. Avoid anything fried or sautéed, as well as creamy sauces and pastry.
- Ask how the food was prepared; don't go by the menu. For instance, the vegetarian option may sound the healthiest choice but it could still be loaded with saturated fat.
- Choose plenty of vegetables with your main course.
- Choose starchy carbohydrates without added fat as the basis for your meal. Try boiled or baked potatoes instead of wedges, roast potatoes and chips; boiled or steamed rice rather than fried or pilau rice; plain noodles instead of fried.
- Be drink aware. Don't forget the calories in both alcoholic and non-alcoholic drinks can add up. Choose sugar-free drinks or water; alternate these with any alcoholic drinks you're having. Always ask for a jug of water with your meal.
- Pace yourself. Eat slowly and wait until you've eaten your main course before you order a pudding.
- If you'd like something sweet, share a dessert or choose healthier options such as fruit, fresh fruit salad minus the cream, or a fruit-based pudding; sorbet instead of ice cream or custard made with lower-fat milk.
- Don't be afraid to leave what you don't want or don't need.

The 'Mediterranean' way can be factored into any style of cuisine. Your goal should be to select dishes with a high vegetable or salad content, served with a modest amount of fish, chicken, lean meat or vegetarian equivalent in a non-fatty sauce.

Foods from around the world – best choices

Chinese

Starters

- Clear soups such as chicken and sweetcorn rather than fried spring rolls, prawn crackers and any other fried dishes.

Main meals

- Beef, chicken, prawn or bean curd with vegetables or black-bean sauce
- Chicken and fish dishes in chilli, soya or oyster sauce
- Chow mein or vegetable stir fry with boiled or steamed rice.

Indian

Starters

- Grilled poppadums
- Tandoori or tikka dishes.

Main meals

Traditional Indian dishes are heavy on the oil and in some cases on ghee (clarified butter) and coconut cream. If unsure don't be afraid to ask the type of fat used for the dish you're thinking of ordering.

- Chicken or fish dishes based on yoghurt or tomato instead of creamy curries such as korma and passandra
- Dhal (lentil curry – but ask for ones without ghee or butter, often added after cooking for a creamier taste)
- Beans or chickpea (chana) curry

- Vegetable dishes but allow these to cool for a few minutes, then skim the oil layer from the surface and discard it
- Saffron or plain boiled rice
- Indian breads – naan or plain chapattis (without ghee or butter) instead of filled varieties (keema and peshwari).

Traditional Indian desserts are high in fat and sugar, so go for the sorbet option or a fruit salad.

Italian

Starters

- Bread sticks or plain crusty bread
- Melon with Parma ham
- Vegetable soup without cream
- Vegetable entrée, such as asparagus with a little parmesan cheese or ham (without melted butter)
- Garden salad with the dressing on the side.

Main meals

- Pasta with tomato-based or seafood sauces, e.g. arrabbiata sauce, Napolitana, primavera and so on; avoid creamy sauces
- Choose thin-crust pizza with vegetable toppings, ham, chicken, seafood and Hawaiian. Add extra vegetable toppings
- Ravioli with ricotta and spinach.

By planning ahead and making healthier choices you can enjoy eating out with friends and family and still manage your cholesterol levels.

In this chapter we have explained why making small changes to your diet over time can help you towards your goal of lowering your cholesterol and improving your heart health. There is a lot to consider in Step 2 of our cholesterol-lowering plan and you may find it easier to tackle the cardio-protective diet first and then go on to maximising our 'cholesterol busters'. By making a few small changes and building these up over time you can achieve significant cholesterol lowering. But take it at your own pace. You will probably want to revisit this chapter again and again to refresh your memory on its contents. Don't forget to make the most of our handy tools and tips including keeping a food diary, planning ahead and checking out our meal planner, healthy shopping list and heart-healthy recipes.

CHAPTER 8

Step 3: Exercise and de-stress

Now that you have a better understanding of cholesterol, and are familiar with all the dietary approaches to lowering it, this step focuses on physical activity and controlling your stress levels.

It is amazing to think that regular physical activity can cut the risk of developing most major chronic diseases, lengthen your life and make you happier, more confident, and improve your shape and size.

Even if you've never exercised before, you can find ways to add physical activity to your day. Once exercise is a normal part of your routine, you'll wonder how you ever did without it. If exercise is new for you, don't forget to check with your doctor or cardiac rehabilitation nurse before starting a new exercise plan. This is especially important if you haven't exercised for a long time, have had a heart attack or have episodes of angina, or if you think you may be at risk of coronary heart disease.

According to the latest figures from Public Health England, physical inactivity is responsible for 1 in 6 (17 per cent) of deaths in the UK. This makes it as dangerous as smoking! Yet over a quarter of us are still inactive, falling short of the recommended 150 minutes of moderate activity each week.

There are many reasons why we are physically inactive. Stressful, busy days and a lack of opportunities to be active are commonplace for many of us. The technical revolution of the last 50 years means that most of us are office-based and sitting for most of the day. Sitting, if we let it, can also dominate our leisure time. It's easy to sit in front of a screen and be entertained, or go for a drink, visit the cinema or have a meal out with friends. We are over-reliant on cars and other motorised forms of transport and at the end of the day all we want to do is sink down in front of the TV.

But managing the amount of physical activity we do and limiting the effect that stressful situations have on our behaviour is the third step in lowering our cholesterol levels. Now is the time to get the whole family active. Just by making activity a normal part of every day from the very moment your children are born means it will naturally become a lifelong healthy habit. So whether it's limiting the time babies spend strapped in their buggies or young children play computer games, finding active pastimes for older adults, or just standing up and moving more, all family members of all ages can benefit from being more active.

Exercise

What kind of physical activity is best?

A complete physical activity routine includes three kinds of activity:

Aerobic exercise is any exercise that uses the large muscle groups in your legs, buttocks and arms. It results in your heart and lungs having to work harder to supply more oxygen to your muscles than is normally needed while resting. After all, your heart is a muscle and it needs to be exercised from time to time. Aerobic exercise helps improve your stamina, strengthen your heart and keep it in tip-top form so it can work more efficiently, pumping blood to every part of your body. Aerobic activities also burn up calories, helping you to control your weight.

For most people, aerobic exercise means activity of light to moderate intensity which should gently increase your breathing and heart rate. One way to tell if you are working at a moderate intensity is that you can still hold a conversation even though you are a bit out of breath.

Examples of aerobic activities

Moderate aerobic workout	More vigorous aerobic workout
Brisk walking (flat surface)	Brisk walking uphill
Jogging (slow)	Running
Cycling	Skipping
Swimming	Team sports such as football
Golf (on foot)	Climbing stairs
Gardening	Racket games such as badminton
Hiking (flat ground)	Hiking (uphill)
Gentle dancing	Salsa/Zumba/Bhangra/ballroom dancing

Daily chores such as shopping, cooking or housework don't count towards your 150 minutes a week. This is because the effort needed to do them isn't hard enough to get your heart rate up.

Resistance training – also called strength training. Resistance training can firm, strengthen and tone your muscles, as well as improve bone strength and help with good posture and balance. Building muscle will help to boost your metabolism, so that you naturally burn more energy when at rest as well as when you are active. Resistance training can help you to maintain a healthy weight, offset bone loss and give you more energy too. Examples include: carrying shopping, walking up stairs or weight and floor training at the gym (e.g., push-ups, lunges, bicep curls, lifting weights).

Flexibility exercises are equally important. These stretch and lengthen your muscles. They help improve joint flexibility, posture, relax your mind and keep muscles supple, thereby preventing injury. Examples include bending and stretching, Pilates, yoga and Tai Chi.

Benefits of exercise

A healthier heart

According to the British Heart Foundation, if you are active, you are less likely to have a heart attack than someone with exactly the same risk factors who is inactive. People who are regularly active have up to 35 per cent lower risk of CHD and stroke than someone who isn't. Almost any kind of physical activity, performed consistently, can strengthen your heart so it pumps with less effort and keeps your artery walls supple, decreasing your risk of heart disease.

If you have had a heart attack, or are at high risk of a heart attack, talk to your GP. At the very least they are likely to advise you to avoid vigorous or high-intensity activities such as sprinting or weight-lifting.

Improved lipid profile

Moderate to intense aerobic exercise (any exercise, such as walking, jogging, swimming or cycling that raises the heart rate for 20 to 30 minutes at a time), at least five times a week, can improve your cholesterol profile by raising your level of HDL cholesterol. Regular exercise can also bring about reductions in LDL cholesterol and is believed to prevent the oxidation of LDL cholesterol, a process that encourages it to stick to artery walls.

Recent evidence suggests that the duration of exercise, rather than the intensity, is the more important factor in raising HDL cholesterol, but both duration and intensity have been shown to be beneficial. Becoming more physically active through regular aerobic exercise can increase HDL cholesterol by about 5 per cent within two months, and can improve LDL-cholesterol levels and lower triglycerides too. If you have raised triglycerides, 150 minutes per week of moderate intensity activity over several weeks could lower them by as much as 20–30 per cent.

Better blood pressure control

No matter what your age, weight or gender, exercise is good for helping to lower blood pressure. Studies have shown that on average, those that did regular aerobic exercise reduced their systolic blood pressure by nearly 4 mmHg, and their diastolic blood pressure by more than 2.5 mmHg. But experts caution that those with high blood pressure should avoid any activity that is very intensive such as sprinting or weight-lifting. These kinds of exercises will quickly raise your blood pressure, and put unwanted strain on your heart and blood vessels.

Less risk of diabetes and better diabetic control

Exercise can help prevent or delay type 2 diabetes in a number of ways:

- By helping with weight loss.
- By increasing insulin sensitivity. Improved insulin sensitivity just means that your body is more responsive to the insulin that it produces. It's a good thing.

If you are already a diabetic, research shows that both aerobic exercise and resistance training can help control diabetes. The greater benefit comes from a programme that includes both. People who are newly diagnosed with type 2 diabetes, and those at risk of developing it, are encouraged to adopt a regular programme of physical activity with the aim of reducing their symptoms or preventing progression to diabetes.

Compliance with these types of programmes can result in significantly better health outcomes.

Weight control

Exercise can help maintain a normal healthy weight, prevent excess weight gain and help maintain weight loss. The more intense the activity, the more calories you burn.

Reduced cancer risk

If you exercise regularly, you stand a good chance of reducing your risk of cancer of the lung, breast, prostrate, uterus, and bowel when compared to those that don't exercise. The exact mechanisms are not clear but it may be due to keeping weight down and stress levels low.

Improved mood

Physical activity can trigger the production of endorphins, natural chemicals which can leave you feeling happier and more relaxed. As exercise tones and improves your shape you may also feel better about your appearance, which can boost your confidence and improve your self-esteem.

Strengthens bones and improves joint structure and joint function

Your bones grow stronger with exercise, particularly with resistance training, and high-impact activities such as jogging or jumping. These weight-bearing exercises also help lower your odds of getting osteoporosis or brittle bones as you grow older, especially when combined with a healthy diet and sufficient vitamin D.

How much is enough?

Adults should aim for at least 150 minutes of moderate intensity aerobic activity each week. For instance, this could be 30 minutes a day, five days a week. Each bout of activity needs to be at least 10 minutes. If you're not used to being active, start slowly and gradually build up to 150 minutes every week.

Being active for longer increases health benefits. For the best results, you should also do activities that will strengthen your muscles such as resistance training, lifting and carrying at least twice a week.

What's stopping you?

Do any of these excuses sound familiar? Try turning the negative into a positive.

'Exercise takes too much time'

Exercise does take some time, but there are ways to make it manageable. Plan your exercise so it becomes part of your daily routine. Make your daily physical activity a priority in your schedule. If you don't have 30 minutes in your day, try to find three 10-minute periods.

'Exercise tires me out'

You might feel a little tired when you initially start your programme but once you have established a regular routine, you're likely to have even more energy than before. As you progress, daily tasks will seem easier. And you'll feel more relaxed afterwards.

'I am too old to exercise'

You are never too old to exercise! No matter what your age, you can always find an activity that is suited to your particular fitness level. Most people become less physically active as they age, but keeping fit is important throughout life.

'You have to be athletic to exercise'

Most activities don't require any special athletic skill. For example, brisk walking is a great heart-healthy activity. Others include swimming or cycling, as long as they're done at a pace that increases your heart and breathing rate.

'Exercise is expensive'

You don't have to join a gym to exercise. Lifestyle activities, like going for a brisk walk or jog, or using bags of sugar or cans of food as weights at home are all free.

We can all find reasons to avoid being active. If something is stopping you, try and work out what you can do to get over that barrier.

Choosing the right activity

The key to a successful exercise programme is choosing an activity, or activities, that work well for you. Do what you enjoy or what fits into your lifestyle. Several studies have found that people who add 30 minutes of activity into their day – even the most mundane types of activity, such as gardening or stair climbing – over time reap the same cardiovascular and weight-loss benefits as those who take part in structured programmes.

Look at the following questions to ask yourself, to identify activities you're likely to stick to.

1. Do you prefer to be active on your own, or with others?

Some people lean towards individual activities such as swimming or going to the gym, whereas others find exercise is more fun when they do it with a friend. If you prefer to do your activity by yourself, it can be more challenging to maintain your momentum and motivation. Whereas if you get a partner, on days when your motivation is low, you are more likely to stick with the programme to avoid disappointing your exercise partner.

2. Do you prefer to be active outdoors or in your home?

Exercise DVDs, bench stepping, skipping or running on the spot allow you to get a good workout, offer shelter from bad weather and the convenience of not having to step beyond your front door. If you enjoy the great outdoors, walking, hiking or hill-walking can be enjoyed at any fitness level. Outdoor activities can be hampered by bad weather so consider choosing a second activity that you can do at home or in a gym.

3. Would you like to join a gym or work with a fitness expert?

It can be expensive, but some people find that regularly going to a gym or working with a fitness trainer helps them to stay more motivated. A personal trainer will help you set goals, design a fitness programme just for you, and help you vary your routine to keep it challenging.

4. Do you like music?

If so, sign up for classes in line dancing, flamenco, Zumba, Bhangra, folk or Scottish dancing. All provide a terrific workout and a lot of fun. Or listen to music while you exercise; your favourite tunes can set the pace for your activity and make the time go faster.

Tips to stay safe

- Wear comfortable shoes that give you good support and choose clothes that allow free movement. Stretchy materials and elastic waistbands are ideal. Dress in layers, especially if you are exercising outdoors, so that you can remove your outer garments as you warm up.
- Do some stretching exercises both before and after your activity to help avoid pulling a muscle or experiencing muscle stiffness the following day.
- Keeping hydrated is important before, during and after exercise to prevent dizziness, cramps and exhaustion. Drink a large glass of water at least 20 minutes before your workout and while you exercise sip from a water bottle as and when you feel like it. Do not wait until you are thirsty to drink; by then you are already dehydrated. Have another glass of water after your workout.
- Start slowly and build up the length and pace of your activity gradually.
- The Golden Rule: always stop if you're in pain, feel dizzy or unwell.

Choose your hour

People who work out in the morning are most likely to stick with a routine. But if you are not a morning person, your best time is whenever works for you.

Creating opportunities

It's easier to stay physically active over time if you take advantage of everyday opportunities to move around. With some creative thinking there are ways to build exercise into a busy lifestyle. It is good to aim for around 10,000 steps a day but most people only manage around 2000–3000. A pedometer will help you monitor just how many steps you take each day.

Find out how much you are doing now and then decide how you can increase it. You can use some of the options below:

- Use the stairs, both up and down, instead of the lift or escalator. Start with one flight of stairs and gradually build up.
- Park a little distance away from the office or shops and walk the rest of the way. If you take public transport, get off a stop or two early and walk.
- Walk your children to and from school. This will also help them develop a pattern of physical activity. If parents are physically active, their children are likely to follow their example and be active too.
- Young mums can set up a buggy group with other mums and go on long walks with the children.
- Avoid sitting down for long periods. Take frequent activity breaks when watching TV, at your workstation, or when at the computer. Get up and stretch, walk around, and give your muscles and mind a chance to relax.
- Instead of eating that extra snack in your break, take a brisk stroll around the neighbourhood or your office building.
- Do more structured exercise during your lunch break. Does your office have a gym, or arrangements with a local gym or nearby swimming pool?
- Plug the phone in upstairs so that you have to climb a flight of steps to answer it or make a call.
- Stand while talking on the telephone.
- Do housework and gardening at a more vigorous pace. Consider using a push-mower instead of an electric or motor mower in the garden.
- Offer to give a neighbour's dog a long, brisk walk every day.
- Stop using online shopping and banking services and instead go to the supermarket, shopping centre or bank in person to do your chores.
- Keep moving while you watch TV. Lift hand weights, or pedal an exercise bike. Better still – turn off the TV and take a brisk walk.

- Make your social life more active. For example, swap nights out in the pub or at a restaurant for dancing or ten-pin bowling.
- Turn exercise into a fun family event. Have a game of football or Frisbee in the park, or pack up a picnic and go for a walk in the country.
- Walk to the shops for your daily newspaper rather than taking the car or having it delivered.

Set some goals

Setting some short-term goals will get you on the right track to achieve that long-term goal. Keep the SMART (specific, measureable, attainable, realistic and time-orientated) principle in mind. (See chapter 6.)

If your goal is to walk an hour a day, five days a week, you may want to set several interim short-term goals along the way. A good short-term goal might be to walk for three 10–minute sessions on Tuesdays, Thursdays and Saturdays. Whatever your short-term goals are, write them down. Then gradually increase the number of minutes you spend and the number of days a week you walk until you reach your overall goal. Once you've reached that goal, you can think about the next one.

Fill in an activity diary to see what you're doing and how much of it counts towards your 150 minutes a week target.

Example of a personal activity diary

Day of the week	Type of moderate intensity activity	Time spent doing each activity	Total time spent being active each day
Monday	Nothing		0 minutes
Tuesday	Aerobics class in the gym	45 minutes	45 minutes
Wednesday	Nothing		0 minutes
Thursday	Brisk walk	15 minutes	15 minutes
Friday	Dancing	20 minutes	20 minutes
Saturday	Sweeping Vacuuming	10 minutes 20 minutes	30 minutes
Sunday	Brisk walk	20 minutes	20 minutes

Look back at your completed personal activity diary. How did you do?

If you were active for 30 minutes or more only on two days of the week, set yourself a higher target for the following week. Think how you can build in more physical activity on the days you are less active.

Staying active is a big challenge. Here are some tips to help you keep going:

- Use your activity diary to help you plan ahead and set new goals
- Use a pedometer; it's an excellent way to keep track and to motivate you to stay physically active
- Do things you enjoy or that are easy to fit into your routine
- Be creative and vary your activities
- Get your friends and family involved
- If you miss a day just start again tomorrow
- Remember how being active will help to make you feel healthier, more energised, toned and self-confident.

Summary

- Being physically active can
  - help you improve your cholesterol levels
  - help reduce the risk of a range of health conditions including coronary heart disease
  - help you maintain a healthy weight
  - help you lose excess fat around your waist
  - improve your self-esteem and confidence
- Always choose activities you can enjoy or fit easily into your lifestyle
- Every 10 minutes of moderate intensity activity counts
- Set realistic SMART goals
- You can monitor your activity by using an activity diary, step counter or an electronic app on your phone.

Stress

What is stress?

Stress is a state of mind, not an illness, so it is difficult to obtain a precise definition or measure of it. 'Stress' is a word people often use to describe how they feel when everything seems too much. We all experience and react to stress in different ways. It's a normal part of modern life. When your stress levels are high, your mood and performance can suffer and if this goes on for too long it can become a real problem and affect your health. The good news is you can learn to manage your stress by adopting new healthy coping mechanisms.

The stress mechanism

When faced with a stressful situation, hormones such as adrenaline and cortisol are secreted into the bloodstream. This causes the heart rate to increase, raises blood pressure, increases blood flow to the muscles and allows more air to enter the lungs. This 'fight-or-flight' reaction is nature's way of channelling our resources to help us escape from immediate danger. However, typical modern-day difficulties, such as money worries, work deadlines and relationship problems, also trigger the stress response. It's not normal to fight or run from these types of stresses so there is no immediate 'release' and recovery from the stress. As a result, hormone levels continue to build and can be detrimental to our health.

What are the signs of stress?

Listen carefully to your body, since stress can express itself in many ways. Here are a few common examples:

Physical signs: dizziness, general aches and pains, difficulty sleeping, tiredness, weight gain/loss, racing heart, tight, knotty feelings in your stomach, indigestion, frequent coughs and colds.

Mental signs: constant worry, difficulty in making decisions, lack of concentration.

Emotional signs: sudden bursts of anger, anxiety, tearful, frequent mood swings, sense of hopelessness.

Stress and heart disease

There is limited evidence to suggest that stress contributes to coronary heart disease or heart attacks. But if you have coronary heart disease and are under a lot of stress, it may bring on symptoms of angina. More research is needed to determine how stress contributes to heart disease.

One way stress can affect your health is by affecting your lifestyle, your behaviour and your coping mechanisms. Some people may choose to unwind with a drink or two; others by snacking or with a cigarette. When these coping mechanisms regularly replace healthy behaviours, or when stress affects your motivation to eat well or your exercise routines, it starts to affect your health. Over time this change in health behaviour can contribute to the development of cardiovascular risk factors.

Tips to de-stress

- Keep a diary for a few weeks. Recording when and how you experience stress and how you respond to it will help you to recognise patterns and take appropriate action.
- Share your worries or concerns with someone who is either a good listener or who may be able to advise you. As the saying goes, 'a problem shared is a problem halved'.

- Take charge of your time. Don't rush around: take your time and plan what you are going to do and follow it through.
- Practise being more assertive. If people are asking too much of you, be prepared to tell them how you feel and to work with them to find a solution.
- Sell yourself to yourself. When you are feeling overwhelmed, remind yourself of what you do well. Be positive.
- Set realistic goals and expectations. Cut your to-do list in half by deciding what is most important or urgent. Leave less important tasks for another day. It's healthy to realise you cannot do everything all at once.
- Avoid the hustle and bustle of commuting and crowded trains, buses and roads if you are able to. If you can, try leaving for work earlier or consider walking instead.
- Get moving. Virtually any form of exercise from aerobics to team games, jogging or yoga can act as a stress reliever. Being active can boost your feel-good endorphins and distract you from daily worries. Exercise can also improve your sleep, which is often disrupted by stress.
- Learn how to relax. Relaxation is more than just sitting back and being quiet. You should include activities that help you relax in a healthy way in your everyday routine. Take time for yourself. Immerse yourself in a hobby you enjoy. Outdoor activities such as bird watching and gardening can be especially therapeutic.
- Change your lifestyle in a positive way. Smoking, drinking and eating unhealthily are not good ways to deal with stress. If you need help to cope, ask for it.
- Practise optimism! Always try to look on the bright side; focus on the positive things that happen each day, however small or trivial they might be, rather than life's problems.

If you feel you cannot manage your stress levels, don't be afraid to ask for help from a health professional. Talk to your GP as they may be able to help or refer you to a qualified counsellor, psychotherapist or psychologist.

Summary

- Stress is a normal part of life. Some people can cope with a lot and others not.
- If you are affected by excess stress this may result in coping mechanisms that affect your health, such as smoking, excess drinking, unhealthy snacking or more sedentary behaviour (TV viewing, computer gaming).
- Look for stress warning signs and work on the triggers causing you to feel stressed.
- Develop techniques, routines and pastimes that help you to relax and unwind.
- Don't be afraid to ask for help from a professional.

CHAPTER 9

Step 4: Medication

N
ot everyone needs to take a medicine to lower their cholesterol, but for some people it is a vital part of maintaining their health and well-being and helps protect them against future cardiovascular disease.

When will I need to take a medicine?

If you started this journey as a result of advice from your doctor, dietitian or practice nurse, chances are they will be keen to see how you are getting on and discuss the changes you have made to your diet and lifestyle. At your appointment they will want to repeat your cholesterol and blood pressure measurements and will discuss the longer-term management of your cholesterol levels. They will want to determine if your cardiovascular risk (the risk of having a stroke or heart attack) has gone down enough or whether further action needs to be taken to safeguard your health. Your doctor is more likely to suggest you take a cholesterol-lowering medicine in these circumstances:

- Your LDL cholesterol, TC:HDL ratio or Lpa levels are high
- You have been exposed to high cholesterol for a long period of time
- You have a high risk of developing cardiovascular disease before you reach 65 or in the next 10 years if you are older than 65
- You have existing heart disease or diabetes

- Close family members have type 2 diabetes, very high cholesterol or early heart disease
- If any diet and lifestyle changes you have made have not reduced your risk sufficiently.

This appointment is your opportunity to have a meaningful, frank and open discussion with your doctor about the benefits of taking a cholesterol-lowering medicine. It's a chance to air any concerns you might have and to ask how your treatment will be monitored in the long term. Write down any questions you might have before your appointment so you can remember to ask them. If you are on other medications or already in poor health, ask about the likely effects on your health from taking another medicine. It's your choice whether you take a medicine or not, but make sure you have all the relevant information before deciding.

Some people when prescribed a medicine think they no longer have to take good care of their diet or lifestyle. This is not the case: it is still very important to take your diet and lifestyle very seriously.

The importance of taking diet and lifestyle changes seriously

If you are taking a cholesterol-lowering medicine or treatment	If you are not taking a cholesterol-lowering medicine or treatment
Diet and lifestyle changes remain very important because:	Diet and lifestyle changes remain very important when:
• Together with medicines they increase your cholesterol-lowering potential • Following a healthy diet and lifestyle means your medicine has to do less work and may mean your doctor can keep your statin dose lower • A healthy diet and lifestyle has many other health benefits, other than lowering cardiovascular risk • Some people may be less responsive to the effects of cholesterol-lowering medications and therefore lifestyle changes are even more important	• Treatment options are not suitable for medical reasons, not tolerated or don't lower your cholesterol sufficiently • When you are trying for a baby, pregnant or breastfeeding and have to stop taking your normal treatment • If you choose not to take a cholesterol-lowering treatment • When you are not eligible to take a cholesterol-lowering medicine but your cholesterol is high

Cholesterol-lowering medications

Cholesterol-lowering medications have been available to a large number of people for many years and have been shown to be very effective in helping to lower the risk of developing angina or having a stroke or heart attack. They work by lowering the circulating levels of LDL cholesterol and in some cases triglycerides too.

All medicines have the potential to cause side effects, and while these medicines are well tolerated by most people, some individuals may experience problems when taking them. Generally speaking, the older you are, the more medicines you take, and the poorer your health the more likely you are to experience the side effects of any medicine.

Here we introduce the main types of cholesterol-lowering drug, describe how they work and when they might be prescribed. Despite there being a number of cholesterol-lowering drugs, most GPs are only able to prescribe the first of these – a statin. Other cholesterol-lowering drugs are usually only prescribed by specialists with the necessary expertise in treating conditions such as lipid disorders or diabetes.

Your doctor will monitor any cholesterol-lowering medications you are prescribed by routinely checking your cholesterol levels, usually after three months and then routinely every year. For most people the aim is to lower your cholesterol by around 40 per cent, but this will differ from person to person. Ask your doctor about target cholesterol levels when you see them for your routine follow-up appointment.

Statins

Statins are a group of medicines that are very good at lowering LDL cholesterol. Because they are so effective they are usually prescribed in preference to other drugs. Statins work by slowing down the production of cholesterol in the liver by partially blocking the actions of a key enzyme – HMG CoA Reductase.

Because your liver is then less able to make cholesterol, it has to take more LDL cholesterol out of the blood. It does this by making more LDL receptors on the surface of liver cells. These act as little arms, catching the LDL-cholesterol particles and bringing them into the cells where the cholesterol can be broken down for use as bile acids, an essential part of the digestive juices that help break up fats during digestion.

The LDL-cholesterol-lowering effect from statins is gradual, and takes about four weeks to build up from the time you start taking them. Statins are not a cure for high cholesterol, only a treatment, so you will need to continue to take them to maintain the cholesterol-lowering benefits. How much a statin lowers your LDL cholesterol will depend upon the strength (potency) of the statin you are prescribed and the dose at which it is given. You should expect to lower your cholesterol by 20–50 per cent dependent on whether you are taking low-, medium- or high-intensity (sometimes called potency) statin treatment.

Categories of statin treatments

- 20–30 per cent cholesterol lowering – low-intensity/potency
- 30–40 per cent cholesterol lowering – medium-intensity/potency
- 40–50 per cent cholesterol lowering – high-intensity/potency

Statins also have anti-inflammatory properties. It means they help to stabilise existing fatty deposits in the artery wall. This is especially important where these deposits, or plaques, are 'vulnerable' because this type of deposit is more likely to burst. If this happens it could result in a heart attack or stroke.

There are five statins currently licensed for use in the UK. The drug names are (in order of potency – lowest to highest) fluvastatin, pravastatin, simvastatin, atorvastatin and rosuvastatin.

Dose (mg per day)	Percentage reduction in LDL cholesterol you can expect				
	5 mg/day	10 mg/day	20 mg/day	40 mg/day	80 mg/day
Fluvastatin			21	27	33
Pravastatin		20	24	29	
Simvastatin		27	32	37	42
Atorvastatin		37	43	49	55
Rosuvastatin	38	43	48	53	

Most people today are prescribed either atorvastatin or simvastatin. Neither drug is protected by patent so both can be made and sold fairly cheaply. NICE guidelines published in 2014 recommend 20 mg of atorvastatin as a starting prescription.

Can statins cause side effects?

It is possible for any drug to cause an unwanted side effect, but in large clinical trials, where statins were tested against a dummy drug, the level of side effects reported was equal for both the statin and the dummy pill, suggesting that statins have low levels of side effects. The studies were blinded, meaning that no one (patient or doctor) knew who was getting the statin and who received the dummy pill.

Of course, the types of people that participate in clinical trials are carefully chosen and it is possible that certain characteristics or risk factors may make some people more susceptible to developing side effects when taking a statin. These might include:

- Increasing age or fragility
- Liver or kidney problems
- Any form of existing muscle disease
- Thyroid conditions such as hypothyroid
- High alcohol consumption
- Taking several other medications
- Having a low vitamin D intake
- Consuming grapefruit juice (simvastatin, atorvastatin and lovastatin only).

The government body that regulates the safety of medicines estimates that each year about 2 in every 1,000 people who take statins will experience mild muscle pain. Muscle pain is most likely in the first three months of treatment.

Very rarely, some people taking statins have developed abnormal muscle breakdown, which can lead to kidney problems and be life-threatening. The same safety regulator has estimated that this might happen in 1 or 2 in every 100,000 people who take statins each year.

If you notice any side effects, such as unexplained muscle pain, tenderness or weakness that you think might be related to your statin, it is best to report these to your doctor. He or she can test the levels of your liver enzymes to see if these are raised, which could indicate a problem.

The most commonly reported side effects are minor muscle problems. It is important to understand that the muscle-related pain that is usually associated with statins is more of a generalised muscle pain, a little like what you might experience if you get the flu. Other problems that have been reported are sleep disturbances and gastrointestinal upsets. The vast majority of statin-related side effects are completely reversible once the medication is stopped. It is usually best to speak to your doctor before discontinuing your statin, unless you are experiencing severe side effects.

There has been some concern that there is slightly greater risk of developing diabetes if you take a statin than if you don't. However, it is likely that anyone developing diabetes when on a statin was already at risk from diabetes. The protective effect that a statin gives is still thought to outweigh the negative effects of becoming diabetic.

What can be done if you are experiencing side effects?

If there is reason to suspect your statin is linked to any symptoms that you are experiencing, your doctor may take you off the medication to see if the symptoms disappear and then reappear once the statin is re-started. Different statins are broken down in different ways in the body so if you do not tolerate one you may tolerate another perfectly well. It is also possible to lower the dose or the frequency with which you take a statin so you still receive some benefit.

Ezetimibe

This drug works by blocking the absorption of cholesterol (from cholesterol-rich bile salts and dietary cholesterol) into the body during digestion. It is often given on top of a statin when extra cholesterol lowering is needed but it can be given alone if statins are not tolerated or in people who do not respond to statin treatment. The cholesterol-lowering potential of ezetimibe is lower than that of statins, usually about 10–20 per cent, and there can be significant variation from person to person.

Resins

Sometimes called bile acid sequestrants these drugs were available before statins. Similar to ezetimibe, they work in the gut and bind on to bile acids to stop them being reabsorbed into the body and then recycled. Once bound to resins they leave the body with the faeces. As a result more cholesterol has to be taken out of the bloodstream to replace the lost bile acids.

Resins come in different forms, either as powders, granules or as tablets, and should be taken immediately before or during each meal. The powders and granules have to be mixed with water or fruit juice and can make you feel pretty full. Because resins are not absorbed directly into the body they can be taken during pregnancy or by young children. While they have a good safety record they can cause gastrointestinal side effects, such as stomach upsets, wind and abdominal discomfort and in some cases diarrhoea or constipation. They also raise triglycerides so are not used for people who have both raised cholesterol and triglycerides. They lower cholesterol by about 10–20 per cent.

Fibrates

These are usually prescribed when both LDL cholesterol and triglycerides are raised. They act by reducing the production of a lipoprotein called Very Low-density Lipoprotein (VLDL), which is rich in triglycerides and is produced in the liver. Fibrates also have a modest HDL-cholesterol raising effect. They may be prescribed alongside a statin. The most frequent side effects with fibrates include gastrointestinal discomfort, nausea, headache and skin rash. There are a number of fibrates available and they can lower triglycerides by around 50 per cent and cholesterol by 25 per cent.

Deciding whether to take a medicine

Some people have very strong personal views about whether they want to take a medicine or not, especially if they have no obvious signs of illness and the drug needs to be taken for the rest of their lives.

Taking a statin, or other cholesterol-lowering treatment, will reduce your risk of heart disease and stroke, but it may not prevent a stroke or heart attack from happening. It is also possible, especially if you are vulnerable to side effects, that taking a cholesterol-lowering treatment may affect your quality of life.

In most situations you do not have to make the decision immediately, so take a few weeks to think it through before deciding. Use the time to talk to health professionals, your partner, friends and family. Remember, if you suffer a heart attack this can have a devastating effect not only on you but also on family life and close family members, especially if it results in disability or even death.

If you have had a cardiovascular risk assessment or NHS health check, your doctor or nurse may have talked to you about your risk of suffering an event such as a heart attack or stroke in the next 10 years. Your risk is generated as a percentage: 10 to 20 per cent represents moderate risk and over 20 per cent high risk. This percentage risk is generated by a computer algorithm which is based upon the outcomes of a very large number of patients who were studied over time.

So if your doctor tells you that you have a 10 per cent risk of having a stroke or heart attack in the next 10 years, this means that of 100 people with the same 10 per cent risk, 10 of them will go on to have a stroke or a heart attack in the next 10 years if they are not treated. Treating all 100 people with the same 10 per cent risk level with a statin will mean that only six will go on to have a heart attack or stroke in the same 10-year period. So taking a statin is not a guarantee; it cannot prevent all heart attacks and strokes but it makes them less likely. As the percentage risk increases more people can be spared a heart attack or stroke by being treated with a statin. The table below gives further detail.

Number of heart attacks or strokes prevented, over 10 years, if 100 people with the same risk level take a statin

Percentage risk over 10 years, as assessed by a cardiovascular risk assessment	10%	15%	20%	25%	30%	35%	40%
What this means	Moderate risk		High risk			Very high risk	
Number of people who do not have a heart attack or a stroke (but would not have done so anyway if not taking a statin	90	85	80	75	70	65	60
Number of people saved from having a heart attack or stroke	4	6	7	9	11	13	15
Number of people who have a stroke or heart attack	6	9	13	16	19	22	25

The percentages shown in the table are only based on 10 years of statin usage. Taking a statin for longer than 10 years will continue to afford you protection against a heart attack or stroke.

The future – new cholesterol-lowering medicines

There are a number of promising cholesterol-lowering medications that have recently become available or are well advanced in clinical research trials. Dependent upon the outcome of these studies, and the granting of a licence for use in Europe and approval by NICE in the UK, it is likely that these drugs will become available for prescription.

At first these treatments will be more expensive than statins so it is likely that statins will remain the preferred drug for some time.

However, in the near future, some people will start to benefit from these new drugs. It is more likely that these drugs will be prescribed for:

- People who are at high risk of cardiovascular disease but who cannot tolerate a statin
- Individuals for whom a statin does not work or a statin is not suitable for medical reasons
- People who need combination therapy, for example, where additional cholesterol-lowering on top of a statin is needed.

Treatments for people with Homozygous FH (HoFH)

Lomitapide

Lomitapide is sold under the brand name Lojuxta® and is licensed for use in the UK but, because of the high cost of the drug, it is not currently routinely available. It is made in capsule form to be taken by mouth and is licensed for use in adults with HoFH (homozygous FH). HoFH is an inherited high cholesterol condition affecting around one in every million births. It occurs when a child inherits an altered FH-causing gene from each parent. Provided the treatment plan is followed carefully, Lojuxta has been shown to lower cholesterol by 50 per cent and can help people with HoFH achieve their cholesterol targets.

People taking Lojuxta need to follow a very low-fat diet, usually less than 40–50 g of fat per day for women or 50–60 g of fat per day for men. Most people consume around 70–90 g of fat per day.

Mipomersin

Mipomersin is a new drug. It has the potential to lower LDL cholesterol by more than 25 per cent in people with HoFH. It is given weekly by injection. Mipomersin is currently licensed in the United States but unfortunately not in Europe.

Other cholesterol-lowering medications in development

PCSK9 Inhibitors

Doctors are excited about these drugs, which have recently undergone testing in patient groups under research conditions. They offer potential for many people, including those with FH. They work by preventing the breakdown of LDL receptors, so helping to improve the removal of cholesterol from the blood. They have to be given by injection, but only once every two to four weeks. There are three PCSK9 inhibitors, all of which are in the process of becoming licensed and available for use in the UK.

Cholesteryl Ester Transfer Protein (CETP) Inhibitors

Two Cholesteryl Ester Transfer Protein Inhibitors are currently still in research trials. They have been shown to lower LDL cholesterol and increase HDL cholesterol significantly.

LDL apheresis or lipoprotein apheresis

Apheresis is currently available in the UK, but only for people at very high lifetime risk of cardiovascular disease and for whom a statin is ineffective, not tolerated or does not offer sufficient cholesterol-lowering. It involves regular hospital treatments as an outpatient (usually once every two weeks). The treatment involves passing a person's blood through a dialysis-like machine which filters out unwanted LDL-cholesterol particles. Apheresis is very efficient at lowering LDL cholesterol. Levels return to normal during the weeks between treatments. There are only a small number of centres in the UK that offer LDL-apheresis and currently none in Scotland or Northern Ireland. Consequently people may have to travel significant distances on a regular basis to access treatment.

Summary

- Your doctor may recommend you take a cholesterol-lowering medication. Your doctor's advice will be based on your cholesterol level as well as any other risk factors you have (age, gender, ethnicity, family history, smoking, raised blood pressure, diabetes, etc.).
- It is important to understand why your doctor is advising you to take any medicine, before you take it. It might help to ask about how the medicine would lower your risk, what side effects it might cause, and how often your doctor needs to review your progress on the medicine.
- Statins are the most commonly prescribed cholesterol-lowering drugs and are relatively safe and well tolerated by most people.
- It is more likely that you will experience a side effect on a statin if you are older, have other pre-existing conditions, and/or are on a number of other drugs. If you think you are

experiencing a side effect of your medication, discuss this with your doctor.

- Your doctor or pharmacist can advise if any symptoms you have are likely to be caused by the medicine you are taking. They can advise on alternative treatments or dosing regimes.
- Whether you are on a medication or not it is still very important to look after your diet and lifestyle.

Dietary Supplements

So often people want to know if there is a magic bullet that they can take to lower their cholesterol. There is – it is called a statin! But usually people are looking for a non-medicinal, herbal or natural remedy that can lower their cholesterol and reduce their risk of cardiovascular disease.

Food supplements originally developed from the need to safeguard the intake of key vitamins and minerals. Fortunately, with a few exceptions, most people should be able to get all their vitamins and minerals from eating a healthy and varied diet.

Some sectors of the population however are more vulnerable to dietary deficiency. This is usually for one of two reasons:

1. They have increased nutritional needs from growth (babies, children, adolescents, pregnancy, breastfeeding) or illness (surgery, convalescence, cancer, an inability to absorb sufficient nutrients from the diet).
2. They have a restricted diet, for example, they may have to avoid certain foods because of a food allergy or a medical condition; or they may be on a calorie-controlled diet.

It has been suggested that some supplements and natural herbal preparations have been considered beneficial in reducing cholesterol or cardiovascular risk and these are presented here in this section. Before we come to this it is best to compare the key differences between medicines and dietary supplements as this will help us to understand how and why these products are presented and promoted in the way they are.

Key differences between medicines and dietary supplements

Medicines	Dietary Supplements
All medicines are strictly regulated in the UK and Europe; they have to meet stringent criteria before they can be marketed; medicines have to have a licence for use	Food supplements are less strongly regulated; they are included in food regulations; food supplements are not licensed
Manufacturers of medicines have to operate a system of adverse event reporting direct to the medical regulatory authorities	No formal system of adverse event reporting is legally required although some food supplement companies operate their own scheme
All new medicines intended for human consumption are thoroughly researched to show they are safe and have the desired effect; studies are well designed and in large numbers	Any research on supplements, or their components, is usually (but not always) in smaller numbers of people and of poorer quality While all food should be safe for human consumption there is no obligation to hold clinical research for a specific food supplement
New medicines are protected by patents – allowing the manufacturer some protection against competition from other drug companies for a defined time period – this allows them to recoup the investment in development and clinical trials	Usually no protection is offered against competitors
Manufacturers claims, wording on pack, and advertising where permitted, is highly regulated and has to be approved by the relevant regulatory authorities	There are voluntary schemes that review food supplement advertising and promotion and pack copy but these are not mandatory; claims made on pack are regulated by European food legislation and policed in the UK by Trading Standards and the Advertising Standards Authority
Medicines can make medical claims – to treat, prevent or cure a condition – provided there is sufficient evidence to this effect	Food supplements cannot claim to treat, prevent or cure a condition; they can under certain circumstances claim to reduce a risk factor such as cholesterol or high blood pressure

Medicines	Dietary Supplements
Some medicines can be sold over the counter (GSL), some can be sold only in pharmacies (P) and others only on prescription (POM)*	Dietary supplements are generally widely available and there are no restrictions on purchasing
	Herbal supplements with evidence of use for over 30 years can be marketed under relatively new legislation provided they comply

*GSL: General sales list; P: Pharmacy only; POM: Prescription only medicine

Are dietary and natural supplements safer than medicines?

Most people see dietary supplements as a safer, more natural way of maintaining good health and treating any ailments. But to assume that all dietary and herbal supplements are completely safe can be dangerous. Some supplements are marketed in high doses and some herbal products have potent effects. For example, vitamins A and D and the mineral iron can be toxic in large amounts. In fact, iron poisoning is a common form of accidental poisoning in children. Large amounts of beta carotene taken in two large well-designed studies resulted in higher levels of lung cancer in smokers compared to placebo, but in other equally well-designed studies large doses of beta carotene had no effect on either cancer or heart disease incidence. So when taking a nutrient supplement it is best to stick to one that offers around 100 per cent of the Reference Intake (RI). The RI is the amount that is believed to meet the needs of most adults. Most supplements declare the percentage of the RI they contain on their packaging.

Many naturally occurring chemicals in plants are toxic and can be dangerous if consumed in significant quantities. So herbal and other natural preparations should be taken only after some research, particularly if you are taking a number of other medicines or have underlying health problems. And don't forget to tell your doctor, dietitian or other health adviser all about them. This will help ensure they are best able to advise and look after you.

Below we describe some of the commonly asked about supplements that have a suggested role in lowering cholesterol or maintaining heart health.

Lecithin

Lecithin occurs in a wide range of foods either naturally or as an ingredient because of its emulsifying properties. Its main components are choline (around 25 per cent) and inositol.

Most people have never heard of choline or the phospholipid that is derived from it – phosphatidyl choline. Phosphotidyl choline is closely involved in the metabolism of fats in the body. It is the main phospholipid responsible for the structural integrity of cell membranes where it is found alongside both fatty acids and cholesterol (see image on page 9). It is also required for cholesterol and lipid transport around the body as it helps to stabilise the lipoprotein structures that carry blood fats.

We can make choline ourselves; however, its synthesis is dependent upon our stores of vitamin B_{12} and folate and the speed at which we are able to make it. It is thought that there may be some stages of our lifecycle, such as rapid periods of growth and development, when we are partly dependent upon dietary sources too. Choline is found in foods such as eggs, soy, peanuts and liver, as well as manufactured foods, and dietary intakes can be as high as 1000 mg choline per day. There are no agreed dietary recommendations in the UK or Europe, but in the USA an acceptable daily intake of 550 mg day has been set for adults.

Inositol is believed to be a vitamin-like nutrient too. It is particularly high in cereals with a high bran content, nuts, beans and fruit.

At the moment there is insufficient evidence of a cholesterol-lowering effect of lecithin, choline or inositol.

Vitamin D

Vitamin D will not lower cholesterol levels but it is intimately linked to cholesterol. For this reason it may be worth taking a supplement if you are at risk of low vitamin D status. It is believed that about one fifth of adults and one sixth of children (as many as 10 million people in England) may have low vitamin D levels.

There have been a number of studies that have suggested a relationship between poor vitamin D status, diabetes and cardiovascular disease. As yet there is no proof that low vitamin D status can cause cardiovascular disease; it may just be an indication of a poor diet or lifestyle. However there are ongoing studies which may be able to show a more direct causal effect in due course.

Vitamin D can be made in the body. The first step in the process is the action of ultraviolet (UV) light on cholesterol precursors in skin. This is followed by two further chemical steps, the first in the liver and the second in the kidney. Because of the geographical position on the earth's surface the UK only has enough UV light of the correct wavelength at certain times of the year (April to October). In theory, because we can store excess vitamin D, most of us can make enough vitamin D during late spring, summer and early autumn to last us over the winter. Ideally we should have about 30 minutes of exposure to sunlight between 11 a.m. and 3 p.m. before applying sun cream or face creams that contain UV filters. For most people this short expo- sure should not put them at risk of sunburn. However, especially if you have sensitive skin, it is important not to sit or work in very strong sunshine without adequate protection.

Some groups of the population are more at risk of vitamin D deficiency, either because of the high needs of growth (vitamin D is needed for normal bone growth and develop- ment) or because their skin cannot make enough vitamin D. People aged 65 and above have less ability to produce vitamin D partly due to the skin thinning and a tendency to expose less

skin to sunlight. Other people at risk of low vitamin D deficiency include people with darker skin, women during
pregnancy, children, teenagers, people who are obese and those
who are housebound. Those living in the north of England and
in Scotland are at higher risk than those in the south of England,
the Midlands or Wales.

Lack of vitamin D in children can lead to poor bone growth
and bowing of the long bones (rickets). In adults it can cause
bone pain and osteomalacia. The bone pain experienced with
vitamin D deficiency can mistakenly be attributed to the generalised muscle pain caused by statins. So there may be good
reason to take a regular vitamin D supplement if you are older
than 65, have limited sun exposure, or fall into one of the 'at
risk' groups. Our levels of vitamin D are usually at their lowest
during the winter months so this is another reason to suspect
deficiency at this time of year.

Sadly, we get little vitamin D from food. Vitamin D is only
found in a few foods such as oily fish, egg yolk, fortified dairy
products and breakfast cereals. When choosing a supplement
look for one that contains between 5 mcg and 25 mcg (5–25
µg) of vitamin D per day. There are some vitamin D preparations that are sold as licensed medicines. Where this is the case
the vitamin D levels are usually declared in International Units
(IU). 1 mcg (1 µg) is equal to 40 IU. Medicines often have
higher levels of vitamin D than supplements. There are also
two different supplemental forms of vitamin D – vitamin D_2
and vitamin D_3. Vitamin D_3 appears to have a longer shelf life
(less susceptible to processing and storage losses) and is more
potent than vitamin D_2.

If you don't have two to three portions of dairy products
each day, or the fortified soya alternatives, you might also be
lacking in calcium, so our advice would be to take a combined
supplement. Oily fish (where you eat the bones), sesame seeds,
pulses, hard water direct from the tap and green vegetables all
provide calcium too, but dairy foods usually account for three-
quarters of our intake.

Fish oils

Fish oils can either be obtained from the body of the fish (herring, sardines, anchovies) or from the fish liver (cod, halibut or shark liver oil). Fish oils are rich sources of omega-3 fatty acids as well as vitamins A and in some cases vitamin D too. The very high levels of vitamin A in fish liver oil can be a disadvantage because vitamin A can be toxic and the high levels limit their use. Fish body oils are usually a better bet because they have lower levels of vitamin A and D and higher levels of the important long chain omega-3 fatty acids. The two main long chain omega-3 fatty acids are EPA – eicosapentaenoic acid and DHA – docosahexaenoic acid. These long chain omega-3 fatty acids have been shown to help reduce inflammation, prevent blood clotting and are believed to reduce the risk of cardiovascular disease. (See page 114.)

The best evidence of benefit has come from studies looking at people that have had a first heart attack. In one study, more individuals who were encouraged to eat two portions of oily fish per week, or to take a fish oil capsule, survived the two years following their first heart attack compared to those who did not get this advice. There were no reductions in the number of heart attacks suffered, only that those eating oily fish or fish oil were less likely to die as a result.

More recent studies have failed to reproduce this effect and this may be due to the study design and /or because people in more recent studies were taking a number of other potent medications that could potentially mask any of the beneficial effects on coronary death attributable to fish oils.

Consequently, doctors are no longer able to prescribe licensed fish oil supplements to people after a heart attack. However, advice to eat oily fish is still a key part of the dietary advice given both to the general public and those people at greater risk of heart disease.

Because of possible contaminants in oily fish young girls and women of childbearing age should not eat more than two portions of oily fish per week. Other groups can consume up to four portions per week.

See the advice on page 117 for fish consumption guidelines.

Vitamin A supplements should not be taken by women in the lead-up to or during pregnancy. Other groups should consume no more than 1500 µg of vitamin A per day from both food and supplements. Vitamin A supplements at the beginning of their shelf life are likely to contain more vitamin A than stated on the label to guard against vitamin losses as they age.

Coenzyme Q10

Sometimes known as ubiquinone, coenzyme Q10 can be made in our bodies; but to do so we use a pathway that is also used to produce cholesterol. Coenzyme Q10 is also widely distributed in the food we eat. Rich sources include meat, fish, nuts, rapeseed and soya oils. Smaller amounts are found in vegetables, fruits, eggs and dairy foods.

Statins, the most frequently used of all the cholesterol-lowering drugs, partially block an enzyme (HMG CoA reductase) at a key stage in the production of both cholesterol and coenzyme Q10. This has led to the suggestion that statins may reduce the production of coenzyme Q10 and that low coenzyme Q10 levels might be associated with the muscle aches and pains (myalgia) and muscle conditions like myopathy occasionally experienced with statins. There is a further suggestion that coenzyme Q10 might be beneficial in reducing or preventing these side effects.

A few small studies have been conducted in people with statin-related myopathy with mixed results. So at the present time there appears to be no conclusive evidence of benefit from coenzyme Q10 supplementation in relieving statin-related muscle symptoms.

Although far from proof, there is evidence of benefit from anecdotal stories. So while routine use should not be encouraged or recommended, there may be a case for a trial period of coenzyme Q10 in people at high risk of cardiovascular disease and for whom statins are an important cholesterol-lowering therapy.

The level of coenzyme Q10 in the body tends to decrease with age. Supplements containing between 15 and 60 mg of coenzyme Q10 per day are available.

Garlic

Garlic is a member of the allium family (garlic, onion, leeks and chives) and has been shown to have antibacterial properties. The active ingredient (allicin) is unstable when cooked. One 2–4 g clove of garlic can provide around 5–20 mg of allicin.

Garlic has long been thought to help lower LDL cholesterol. However, much of the research around garlic is in small studies and can be of relatively poor quality. Added to this is the complication that it is not always easy to determine the nature of the garlic supplement being tested and the amount of active ingredient it contains as this may vary from preparation to preparation and from batch to batch.

Scientists in the USA and Malaysia reviewed the available evidence in 2000 and in 2009 respectively. In the first review researchers concluded that the effect of garlic was probably small but also only lasted for a short time, as they could find no evidence of cholesterol-lowering at six months when compared to those taking the placebo. In the second review the authors looked at 13 randomised controlled trials and found no effect on cholesterol levels at all.

Red yeast rice

Red yeast rice is an extract obtained from rice that has been fermented with a yeast called *Monascus purpureus*. It has been used as a natural herbal supplement in China for many years.

There is little doubt that these products do have cholesterol-lowering ability but the quality can vary and the consumer has no way of knowing if the product can be relied upon to have the desired effect. Fermented red yeast rice preparations actually contain Monakolin K, the same active ingredient that is present in Lovastatin, one of the early statins, so it is not surprising that they can cause the same side effects that are reported for lovastatin.

Because these products are not regulated as medicines, the lack of standardised manufacturing practices can lead to significant variation between brands and also from one batch of a named brand to another.

There is also some evidence that a toxin – citrinin – can be present in some preparations and also reports of muscle damage following the use of red yeast rice. One survey of red yeast rice products on the market in 2011 showed that some of them contained very little Monacolin K.

Our best advice is not to use red yeast rice to replace or in addition to conventional medicines, or if you are pregnant, trying to become pregnant, or breastfeeding. If you need to take a statin it is much better for you to be under the supervision of your GP, know the exact dose of statin that you are on and the expected extent of its cholesterol-lowering effect. This will allow you and your doctor to assess your cholesterol reduction and change your medicine if appropriate.

Phytosterols (plant sterols and stanols)

These have been covered in more detail in the section on cholesterol-busting foods. They are commonly added to dairy foods such as milk, yoghurts, 'milk shots' and spreads. However they are also available in supplement form. Generally speaking, dietary supplements that contain phytosterols have been less well researched. While we know that they lower cholesterol by about 7–10 per cent when eaten in quantities of 2–3 g per day within a dairy food, we do not know if they work equally well when consumed as a tablet or capsule.

Dietary supplements of phytosterols often work out cheaper than the fortified food equivalents and therefore can be seen as more attractive. If you do intend to take these it is best to spread the dosage out across the day and always take the supplement with food rather than between meals.

Summary

- Food supplements are not a replacement for selecting healthy foods or for preparing, cooking and eating a healthy balanced diet, but in some cases may have some benefits in those people with higher needs or who are at risk of nutrient deficiency.
- In particular, people at risk of vitamin D deficiency could benefit from taking a regular vitamin D supplement.
- Supplements containing plant sterols and stanols do lower cholesterol, but it is not known if they perform as well as foods fortified with sterols and stanols. If chosen they should be spread throughout the day and taken only with meals. The recommended dose is between 1.5 g and 2.4 g per day. You should not exceed 3 g per day.
- More research into the health effects of garlic, lecithin and red yeast rice is needed before they can be recommended for people wishing to lower their cholesterol levels.
- Health professionals do not currently recommend coenzyme Q10 for people who report statin intolerant muscle-related side effects. Currently there is insufficient evidence of benefit.
- Eating fish at least twice a week, and oily fish at least once a week, is preferred to taking cod liver oil or fish oil supplements. If taking cod liver oil it is important not to take any other vitamin A containing foods or supplements (liver, liver pate, multivitamins, etc.). See our advice on vitamin A intake in the Q&A section at the back of the book.

Recipes

We have developed some tasty recipes that are either naturally low in saturated fat or lower than their equivalents. Each in its own way can play a role in helping you to manage your cholesterol levels, plus many of our recipes contain vegetable proteins like soy and nuts, soluble fibre from fruits, vegetables, beans and peas and oats.

We encourage you to reduce your salt intake and experiment with more herbs and spices to provide lots of flavour. By cooking from scratch and limiting the number and quantity of high-salt ingredients in your cooking, you will already be cutting your salt intake. If you can't do without salt, try switching to a low-salt alternative and choose lower-salt versions of stocks, sauces and gravies where possible.

These recipes are all straightforward to follow and the ingredients are easy to come by and relatively inexpensive.

We recognise there are special occasions when we all want to indulge and for that reason we have included a few ideas like our Surprise Bread and Butter Pudding, our Red Fruit Bomb and our Chocolate Cake and Slow-Cooked Beef Curry. But most of our recipes are deigned to be eaten regularly as part of your weekly routine.

If you need inspiration why not try our two-week planner? It's not intended to be followed to the letter but it does give lots of ideas for the types of meals you might like to try.

Shopping

To make shopping easier and for you to achieve your goals:

1. Write a list. This will make sure you have all the relevant food items and ingredients you need.
2. Never go shopping when you are hungry. An empty stomach may tempt you to buy food you don't want or need.
3. Compare sizes and prices: don't be deceived by bulky packaging.
4. Buy only what you require. Pre-packed items work out dearer if they contain more than you need.
5. Look out for own brands. They are often cheaper and just as nutritious as better-known brands.
6. Money spent on seasonings, herbs and spices is money well spent, as flavours can make food more exciting.
7. Get to grips with food labels to help you compare like-for-like products and make healthier choices – see page 130 on nutrition labels.

Shopping list essentials

- Porridge oats and other oat-based breakfast cereals (check out the sugar content of very processed cereal products)
- Oat bran
- Wholegrain and high-fibre breakfast cereals
- Granary, wholegrain, soya and linseed or rye breads
- Wholemeal pitta bread and wraps
- Brown rice and pasta
- Wholemeal flour
- Fruit, salad and vegetables. As well as those in season, stock up on vegetables that are frozen or canned in water
- Dried fruit
- Unsweetened fruit or vegetable juice
- Extra-lean mince and skinless chicken/turkey

- Fish: fresh or frozen cod, haddock or fresh, frozen or tinned oily fish like mackerel, salmon, pilchards or sardines
- Eggs
- Tinned pulses, e.g., chickpeas, kidney beans, lentils
- Soya products like soya mince, soya nuts, tofu or soya milk
- Unsalted nuts and seeds like sesame, pumpkin and sunflower
- Skimmed, semi-skimmed or 1 per cent fat milk
- Lower-fat cheese. Look out for the words 'reduced fat' or 'light'
- Low-fat, low-sugar yoghurts
- Plant sterol- and stanol-based drinks, yoghurts, spreads and milk
- Unsaturated fats and spreads (e.g., olive, rapeseed or sunflower) – try low fat varieties
- 1 kcal cooking oil spray
- Dried herbs (e.g., basil, oregano, parsley)
- Ground spices (e.g., paprika, cumin, five spice, ginger)

Breakfasts

BREAKFAST GRANOLA

Preparation time: 15 minutes
Cooking time: 30 minutes
Makes 14 portions (60 g each)
Each portion provides 1 g beta glucan

Ingredients

300 g rolled oats
50 g oat bran
½ teaspoon ground cinnamon
¼ teaspoon mixed spice
65 g soft brown sugar

2 tablespoons honey
50 ml rapeseed oil
100 g mixed nuts (such as sliced almonds, chopped walnuts, pecans, macadamia, hazelnuts) chopped into small pieces
100 g ready-to-eat dried apricots, chopped into small pieces
100 g raisins

Method

1. Preheat the oven to 150°C.
2. Combine the oats, oat bran, cinnamon, mixed spice and sugar in a bowl.
3. Mix the honey and oil together and then pour over the oat mixture. Stir to thoroughly coat the oats.
4. Place the mixture on two flat baking trays and bake for 30 minutes.
5. Meanwhile lightly toast the chopped nuts in a thick-bottomed frying pan, taking care not to burn them.
6. Allow the oats to cool, then mix with the nuts and dried fruit and store in a jar or container with a tightly fitting lid.
7. The ingredients may settle so shake before each use to ensure you get a mixture of everything.
8. Serve with cold low-fat milk, low-fat yoghurt or fruit juice.

BREAKFAST MUESLI

Preparation time: 15 minutes
Cooking time: none
Makes 14 portions (62.5 g each)
Each portion provides 1 g of oat beta glucan

Ingredients

300 g rolled oats
50 g oat bran

120 g mixed chopped nuts (such as almonds, walnuts, pecans,
   hazelnuts)
50 g sunflower seeds
50 g pumpkin seeds
100 g ready-to-eat dried apricots, chopped
100 g ready-to-eat dried figs, chopped
50 g dried cranberries
50 g raisins

Method

1. Combine all the ingredients in a bowl.
2. Tip the mixture into a sealed container to keep fresh.
3. The ingredients may settle so shake before each use to
   ensure you get a mixture of everything.
4. Serve with cold low-fat milk, low-fat yoghurt or fruit juice.

BREAKFAST SMOOTHIE

Preparation time: 2 minutes
Cooking time: none
Serves 1 person

Ingredients

1 small ripe banana
80 g frozen fruit (raspberries, blueberries, strawberries,
   blackberries, cherries or a mixture)
150 ml of fruit juice (apple, orange or cranberry)
2 tablespoons (20 g) oat bran

Method

1. Put all the fruit and the oat bran into a smoothie maker or
   food processor.

2. Add the fruit juice and blend to a smooth consistency.
3. Pour into a glass to serve.

HEALTHY KEDGEREE

Preparation time: 5 minutes
Cooking time: 30 minutes
Serves 4

Ingredients

225 g brown rice
1 tablespoon vegetable oil
1 medium onion, diced
1 green pepper, thinly sliced
200 g smoked haddock
100 ml skimmed milk
2 eggs, boiled for 8 minutes, peeled and cut into quarters
1 tablespoon curry paste, or to taste
Black pepper to season

Method

1. Boil the rice in a large pan as per the packet instructions.
2. In a frying pan cook the onion gently in the oil until start-ing to soften, then add the pepper and continue to cook without colouring about 10 minutes in total.
3. Check the haddock and remove any bones. Poach in the milk in a saucepan until just cooked. This should take 4–5 minutes. Take out of the pan and remove any skin. Flake the fish, set aside and keep warm.
4. When the rice is cooked, rinse with hot water, drain and add back to the cleaned pan. Add the curry paste, onion

and pepper mix and seasoning then stir to combine. Lastly add the flaked fish and gently stir.

5. Serve topped with quarters of the boiled egg.

RATATOUILLE, POACHED EGGS AND SAUSAGES

Preparation time: 10 minutes
Cooking time: 30 minutes
Serves 4

Ingredients

2–4 tablespoons oil (olive or rapeseed)
1 large onion, diced
1 clove of garlic finely diced or crushed
1 red pepper cut into 2 cm pieces
1 medium courgette sliced and cut into 2 cm pieces
1 small aubergine cut into 2 cm pieces
400 g can chopped tomatoes
1 teaspoon dried oregano
2–3 tablespoons sun-dried tomato paste
400 ml vegetable stock
Salt and pepper to season 4 eggs
4 vegetarian sausages

Method

1. In a non-stick frying pan, cook the onion and the garlic in 1 tablespoon of the oil for a few minutes until softened but not coloured.
2. Add the pepper, courgette and aubergine and continue to cook for around 5–10 minutes. You may need the extra oil at this stage.
3. Purée the tomatoes with a hand blender if preferred. Add to the pan with the dried oregano, tomato paste and vegetable

stock. Cover and cook on a low heat for around 15–20 minutes until cooked through.

4. Season with salt (if needed) and pepper and keep warm.
5. Meanwhile poach the eggs and grill the vegetarian sausages.
6. Serve the ratatouille with poached egg and a vegetarian sausage.

Cooking Tip Any excess ratatouille can be frozen and used for another breakfast or other mealtime.

For a tasty main meal, try sealing chicken breasts or chicken pieces in a pan with a little oil and then simmering in the ratatouille. Check the chicken is cooked all the way through before serving.

SMOKED SALMON AND SCRAMBLED EGG MUFFINS

Preparation time: 2 minutes
Cooking time: 10 minutes
Serves 2

Ingredients

2 wholemeal English muffins
60 g smoked salmon
A little sunflower spread
2 eggs, beaten and seasoned with black pepper

Method

1. Cut the muffins in half and lightly toast, spread with a little sunflower spread, top with smoked salmon, season and arrange on two plates.

2. Melt 1 teaspoon of sunflower spread in a small non-stick saucepan over a low heat. Add the eggs and stir to gently scramble.
3. Just before the eggs are completely cooked, pour out on top of the muffins (they will continue to cook).
4. Season again with black pepper and serve.

Cooking Tip If you prefer you can poach the eggs instead of scrambling.

STEWED FRUIT

Use as a breakfast on its own, with low-fat yoghurt or to top cereal.
Preparation time: 5 minutes
Cooking time: 10–15 minutes
Serves 4

Ingredients

400 g of fresh fruit (such as apple, apricot, pears, peaches, blackberries, plums, or rhubarb)
50 g sultanas
30–75 g caster sugar (depending upon the sweetness of the fruit you use)
Zest and juice of one lemon
½ cinnamon stick (optional)
2–3 cloves (optional)

Method

1. If using apples or pears, peel the fruit. Wash and cut up the fruit into similar-sized pieces.

2. Combine all the ingredients in a heavy-bottomed saucepan.
3. Cover and cook over a low heat for around 10–15 minutes until the fruit has released some juices and is tender but still holding some shape.
4. Allow the fruit to cool, remove the cinnamon stick and cloves if used.
5. Serve with a few toasted almonds on top.

Cooking Tip This fruit makes a great dessert with low-fat custard, soya cream or low-fat ice cream or topped with our healthy crumble mixture (see page 243)

Instead of fresh fruit, you could use 200 g of stoned dried fruits (such as prunes, figs, dates, apricots or dried apple). You may need to reduce the sugar and add some water to the recipe.

Two ways with porridge:

DATES AND WALNUTS

Preparation time: 2 minutes
Cooking time: 5 minutes
Serves 2

Ingredients

560 ml (1 pint) low-fat milk or fortified soya milk
80 g rolled oats
20 g oat bran
6 dates, chopped
6 walnuts, chopped
1 tablespoon honey (optional)

Method

1. Warm the milk, oats and oat bran in a non-stick saucepan.
2. Add the dates as the mixture comes to the boil, then turn the heat down and simmer until thickened.
3. Serve garnished with chopped walnuts and a swirl of honey.

SPICED APPLE

Preparation time: 2 minutes
Cooking time: 5–10 minutes
Serves 2

Ingredients

1 cooking apple, peeled, cored and diced
1 tablespoon honey
2 tablespoons sultanas
$\frac{1}{8}$ – $\frac{1}{4}$ teaspoon ground cinnamon
560 mls (1 pint) low-fat milk or fortified soya milk
80 g rolled oats
20 g oat bran

Method

1. Cook the apple with the honey, sultanas and cinnamon in a non-stick saucepan until the apple is just tender.
2. In a separate pan, warm the milk, oats and oat bran. Bring the porridge to the boil, turn the heat down and simmer until thickened.
3. Serve topped with the spiced apple.

Cooking Tip You can cook the apple ahead of time and keep in the fridge until needed.

Lunches

GAZPACHO

Preparation time: 40 minutes plus 1 hour chilling time
Cooking time: none
Serves 4

Ingredients

1.2 kg tomatoes
1 large cucumber
1 large red pepper
40 g wholemeal breadcrumbs
2 cloves of garlic
4 tablespoons red wine vinegar
Juice from 2 freshly squeezed oranges
60 ml extra virgin olive oil
2 tablespoons cannellini beans
Salt and pepper to taste

Method

1. To remove the skins from the tomatoes, plunge them into a bowl of boiling water for a few minutes. After a couple of minutes you should be able to easily peel off the skins. It might be best to do this in batches. Cut the tomatoes into quarters and remove any seeds but try to reserve as much of the juice as possible.
2. Peel the cucumber and remove the seeds from the red pepper. Reserve about one-fifth of the tomato, cucumber and pepper for the garnish. Roughly chop the rest of the vegetables and place in a blender with the breadcrumbs, garlic, vinegar, orange juice and two thirds of the oil (in batches if necessary). Blitz until smooth. You can use a little

water to dilute it if necessary but try to use as little as possible. Season to taste.

3. Dice the remaining vegetables finely and reserve with the cannellini beans as a garnish.

4. Gazpacho needs to be served very cold, so chill for at least an hour before serving. Ladle into individual bowls and garnish with the reserved diced vegetables and a swirl of oil.

Serving Tip Serve with wholemeal croutons, chunks of wholemeal bread, or with wholemeal toast.

HERBY LENTIL SALAD

Preparation time: 10 minutes
Cooking time: 2 minutes
Serves 4

Ingredients

2 tablespoons olive oil
1 garlic clove, crushed
4 spring onions, sliced
2 × 400 g (13oz) cans green lentils, drained and rinsed
2 tablespoons balsamic vinegar
3 tablespoons finely chopped herbs (such as parsley, oregano or basil)
125 g (4 oz) cherry tomatoes, halved
½ red chilli, finely diced (seeds removed)
Black pepper

Method

1. Heat the oil in a non-stick pan, add the garlic and spring onions and fry for 2 minutes.

2. Put the lentils, vinegar, herbs and tomatoes in a large bowl.
3. Pour over the garlic and onion mixture, add the chilli, season generously with black pepper and thoroughly mix before serving.

MIXED BEAN AND PEA SALAD

Preparation time: 15–20 minutes
Cooking time: none
Serves 4 as a main dish and 8 as a side salad

Ingredients

200 g of defrosted edamame beans
100 g defrosted frozen peas
½ green pepper, diced
100 g sugar snap peas, blanched for 1–2 minutes
½ can red kidney beans
½ can sweetcorn
100 g cherry tomatoes, halved
100 g cucumber, diced
1 red onion finely chopped

For the dressing

4 tablespoons extra virgin olive oil
Juice of 1 lemon
2 cloves of garlic, crushed
½ teaspoon lemongrass purée
¼ red chilli chopped or ½ teaspoon chilli powder
1 cm grated ginger or ¼ teaspoon ground ginger

Method

1. Combine all the vegetables in a bowl.
2. Mix all the salad dressing ingredients together in an airtight jar.
3. Toss the salad in the dressing shortly before serving.

Cooking Tip Great for packed lunches but pack the dressing separately so the vegetables keep their crunch.

PEANUT AND BANANA TOASTIE

Preparation time: 5 minutes
Cooking time: 5 minutes
Serves 1

Ingredients

2 slices wholegrain bread
2–3 tablespoons crunchy peanut butter
1 large ripe banana, peeled and mashed

Method

1. Lightly toast the bread in a toaster and preheat the grill to its highest setting.
2. Spread the peanut butter on the toast and cover with the mashed banana.
3. Cook for a few minutes under the grill. Keep an eye on it: the banana may brown but don't allow it or any exposed toast to burn.

Cooking Tip Soft fruits, such as banana, plums and peaches, make a great dessert. Just slice, arrange on toast, sprinkle with a little sugar and grill. You can add sliced almonds halfway through cooking. Either eat on its own or serve with a low-fat ice cream or yoghurt.

SPICY MOROCCAN SOUP

Preparation time: 15 minutes
Cooking time: 30 minutes
Serves 4

Ingredients

100 g couscous
1 medium onion, diced
1 small aubergine, diced into 2 cm cubes
1 small sweet potato, diced into 2 cm cubes
2 courgettes, diced into 2 cm cubes
1 large carrot, cut into 1 cm slices
2–3 tablespoons vegetable oil
1 clove garlic, crushed
400 g can of tomatoes
1 litre vegetable stock
2 tablespoons tomato paste
2–3 heaped teaspoons harissa paste
Handful fresh coriander leaves
Handful of fresh mint leaves

Method

1. Place the couscous in a dish, add 100 mls boiling water and set aside.
2. Prepare the vegetables by dicing the onion, aubergine, sweet potato and courgettes into 2 cm pieces. Slice the carrot into 1 cm pieces.

3. In a large heavy-bottomed saucepan heat the oil and fry the aubergine on all sides for a few minutes, allowing it to brown. Add the garlic, onion, courgettes, carrot and sweet potato and cook for 5 more minutes.
4. In a separate dish, blend the tomatoes using a hand blender until smooth and then add to the pan with the stock, tomato paste and harissa paste.
5. Gently simmer until the vegetables are tender.
6. Meanwhile, finely chop a large handful of coriander and mint leaves. Mix these into the couscous.
7. When the soup is ready, divide the couscous equally into bowls and ladle the soup on top.

TOMATO, BASIL AND SOYA BEAN BRUSCHETTA

The little explosions of garlicky tomato goodness make a great lunchtime favourite.
Preparation time: 5 minutes
Cooking time: 5–10 minutes
Serves 2

Ingredients

4 slices wholegrain bread or a small baguette sliced at an angle
2 tablespoons of extra virgin olive or rapeseed oil
50 g frozen soya beans
2 teaspoons vegetable oil
150–200 g cherry tomatoes
1 small clove of garlic, chopped
1 tablespoon of basil, roughly torn or chopped

Method

1. Toast the bread on both sides and then brush with the extra virgin olive oil on one side.

2. Warm the soya beans with the vegetable oil in a small pan until the beans are just starting to thaw.
3. Add the cherry tomatoes and garlic and cook until the tomatoes are softened and starting to release their juices.
4. Add the chopped basil leaves and stir for about 30 seconds.
5. Arrange the bread on plates and top with the tomato and bean mixture.
6. Enjoy while warm.

TUNA NIÇOISE

Preparation time: 10 minutes
Cooking time: 15 minutes
Serves 4

Ingredients

1 × 200 g fresh tuna steak
1 tablespoon olive oil
2 eggs
6 small baby potatoes, boiled, cooled and sliced in half
200 g fine green beans
1 tablespoon extra virgin olive oil
2 tablespoons lemon juice
1 teaspoon wholegrain mustard
200 g cherry tomatoes, halved
⅓ cucumber, sliced
½ red onion, cut in half and finely sliced
100 g mixed lettuce leaves, cut into bite-sized pieces
1 avocado, stoned and diced
1 can of cannellini beans, rinsed and drained
small bunch of fresh herbs such as dill, parsley or basil, roughly chopped
Pepper to season

Method

1. Brush the tuna with the olive oil and season with black pepper. Grill for 8–10 minutes under a low/medium heat, turning once halfway through cooking.
2. Flake the tuna and leave to one side to cool.
3. Boil the eggs in hot water for no more than 8 minutes, leave to cool in cold water, then peel carefully and cut into quarters.
4. Cook the potatoes in their skins by boiling for around 15 minutes, drain and leave to cool.
5. Trim the fine beans and boil for three minutes, drain and plunge into cold water and leave to cool.
6. Make the salad dressing by combining the extra virgin olive oil, lemon juice and grain mustard in a jar and shake until mixed.
7. Toss all the salad items: tomatoes, cucumber, onion, salad leaves, avocado, potatoes and both kinds of beans in the salad dressing and arrange in a large bowl.
8. Arrange the flaked tuna and eggs on top and sprinkle with the chopped herbs and serve.

Main meals

BEEF AND ORANGE CASSEROLE

Preparation time: 20 minutes
Cooking time: 2½ hours
Serves 6

Ingredients

675 g diced lean stewing beef
4 tablespoons plain flour
3 tablespoons rapeseed oil

2 medium onions, chopped
1 clove of garlic, crushed
2 sticks of celery, chopped
2 medium carrots, sliced
2 beef stock cubes, preferably low salt
1 bay leaf
1 sprig of thyme
1 orange
150 g pitted prunes
60 g raisins
Black pepper to season

Method

1. Season the flour with black pepper and toss the diced meat in it to coat it on all sides.
2. Brown the meat on all sides in a non-stick frying pan, in two batches, using one tablespoon of oil each time. Transfer the meat to a large casserole dish.
3. Cook the onions and garlic in the remaining oil. After a few minutes add the celery and carrots and cook for a further 4–5 minutes on a low-moderate heat.
4. Transfer the vegetables to the casserole together with crusty bits remaining in the pan. Add two stock cubes crumbled, bay leaf and thyme and only just cover with hot water.
5. Bring to the boil on the stove and then place in the oven (160°C) for two hours, checking occasionally to make sure there is still enough liquid in the casserole.
6. Meanwhile, place the zest of the orange, together with its juice and the prunes and raisins in a bowl and cover with cling film.
7. After two hours remove the casserole from the oven, add the fruit, juice and zest mixture. Return to the oven for 30 minutes.
8. Serve with fruity, nutty couscous (see following recipe).

Cooking Tip You can cook the casserole up to the end of point 5 the day before you need it.

FRUITY NUTTY COUSCOUS

Preparation time: 20 minutes
Cooking time: 2½ hours
Serves 6

Ingredients

1 medium onion chopped
½ tablespoon rapeseed oil
120 g couscous
50 g mixed nuts chopped
50 g dried fruit of your choice (such as apricots, sultanas)
1 handful of roughly chopped parsley
Black pepper to season

Method

1. Gently fry the onion in the oil for 5–10 minutes until softened but not coloured.
2. Meanwhile chop the nuts, fruit, parsley and prepare the couscous as per the packet instructions.
3. Combine all the ingredients and serve either cold with salad or warm as part of a main meal.

LAMB KEBABS

Preparation time: 15–20 minutes plus time to marinate
Cooking time: 20 minutes
Serves 4

Ingredients for the kebabs

400 g lean lamb, cut into bite-sized pieces
1 large pepper, cut into 16 pieces
2 red onions each cut into 8 pieces
16 chestnut mushrooms
16 cherry tomatoes
8 wooden or metal skewers

Ingredients for the marinade

4 tablespoons olive oil
4 tablespoons fresh lemon juice
Zest of one lemon
Ground black pepper
1 clove of garlic crushed
1 tablespoon of rosemary, finely chopped

Method

1. Make the marinade by mixing all the ingredients together. Use to coat the lamb, cover and leave in the fridge to marinate, ideally overnight.
2. Pre-soak any wooden skewers for 30 minutes.
3. Assemble the skewers with the mushrooms and tomatoes at the ends of each skewer with the lamb, pepper and onion in the centre.
4. Cook under a medium grill or on a barbeque for 15–20 minutes; occasionally basting with any leftover marinade.
5. Serve with fruity, nutty couscous and a green salad.

SLOW-COOKED BEEF CURRY

Preparation time: 30 minutes
Cooking time: 2 hours, or 4+ hours in a slow cooker
Serves 4

Ingredients

1 large onion, chopped
1 clove garlic
3–4 tablespoons rapeseed or sunflower oil
1 inch fresh root ginger, peeled
1 fresh red chilli, finely sliced (seeds included)
1 teaspoon ground turmeric
1 teaspoon lemongrass purée
1 lb lean casserole steak, cut roughly into 2 cm × 4 cm chunks
2 tablespoons of flour, seasoned with black pepper
1 small aubergine or 4–5 baby aubergines (about 200 g)
250 mls soya or oat cream
250 mls water
2 teaspoons tamarind paste
Brown basmati rice to serve

Method

1. Cook the onions and garlic in 1 tablespoon of the oil in a frying pan for a few minutes, without browning. Then add the ginger, chilli, turmeric and lemon grass and continue to cook for another few minutes.
2. When the spiced onions are softened, transfer them to your slow cooker or casserole dish.
3. Toss the beef chunks in the seasoned flour and brown in batches in the remaining oil. Transfer the browned beef pieces to the casserole dish or slow cooker.
4. Slice the aubergine into 1 cm thick rounds, brush with oil, season with pepper and cook under the grill or in the frying pan for a couple of minutes until softened and starting to colour.
5. Add the aubergine, cream and water to just cover the beef, stir and cook gently in the oven (150°C) for 2 hours or in the slow cooker for a minimum of 4 hours. Stir the tamarind paste into the casserole about 30 minutes before serving.
6. Serve with brown basmati rice and a vegetable of your choice.

CASSOULET

Preparation time: 10 minutes plus any soaking time
Cooking time: 3½ hours
Makes 4

Ingredients

350 g canned beans or 185 g dried beans such as pinto or
cannellini beans
2 tablespoons olive oil
4 vegetarian or low-fat sausages
400 g chicken pieces, skinned and fat removed
2 onions, roughly chopped
4 cloves of garlic, crushed or finely chopped
1 large carrot, roughly chopped
1 × 400 g can chopped tomatoes
1 bay leaf
1 teaspoon dried thyme or a large sprig of fresh thyme
3 tablespoons sun-dried tomato paste or 45 g chopped
sun-dried tomatoes
250 ml white wine
2 tablespoons chopped parsley

Method

1. If using dried beans these will need soaking overnight and
   then boiling for 10 minutes before use. Dried beans double
   in weight when soaked.
2. Preheat the oven to 150°C.
3. Heat the oil in a large frying pan. Brown the sausages and
   then the chicken. Set aside.
4. In the same pan cook the onion and garlic for a few minutes
   without colouring. Add the carrot and continue to cook for
   a further few minutes.

5. Pack the beans, meat, cooked vegetables, tomatoes, bay leaf, thyme, tomato paste and wine in a heavy casserole dish. Add enough hot water to just cover the ingredients.
6. Cook in the oven for up to 3 hours, checking the cassoulet about halfway through and adding a little extra water if needed.
7. Add the parsley to the cassoulet just before serving and eat with a chunk of wholegrain bread, essential to mop any juices.

Cooking Tip This is a perfect dish for a slow cooker, but don't forget to boil any dried beans after soaking and before putting in the cassoulet. This is essential to remove harmful toxins in the beans. The canning process also removes the toxins.

CHICKEN AND PRUNE TRAY BAKE

Preparation time: 10–15 minutes
Cooking time: 1 hour
Serves 4

Ingredients:

8 chicken thighs, skin and fat removed
12 prunes, stones removed
400 g baby potatoes, washed but with skins on (cut in half if larger than a golf ball)
2 tablespoons honey
2 tablespoons olive oil
Sprig of fresh rosemary
Juice and zest of 1 orange
2 rashers lean bacon, cut in half lengthways
1 red onion, peeled and cut into 8 wedges
Salt and pepper

Method:

1. Make a large slit in the flesh of the chicken thighs and slip a prune into the middle of each. Place the chicken pieces and potatoes in a large ovenproof dish.
2. Put the honey, olive oil, rosemary, orange juice and zest into a pan and warm through.
3. Wrap the remaining prunes in bacon and place in the dish with the chicken and potatoes.
4. Pour over the warm sauce.
5. Cover loosely with foil and bake in a pre-heated oven at 180°C for 1 hour. You should be left with a sticky sauce in the base of the cooking dish.
6. Arrange the chicken, potatoes and bacon-wrapped prunes on plates. If needed, add extra water to the sauce to loosen then pour over the chicken. Serve with green beans and cauliflower.

Cooking Tip Leave out the potatoes, add cherry tomatoes halfway through cooking and serve with couscous made with chicken stock.

CHICKEN PILAF

Preparation time: 10 minutes
Cooking time: 1 hour 15 minutes
Serves 4

Ingredients

2 tablespoons rapeseed oil
2 chicken breasts, diced
1 onion, diced
150 g pearl barley

¼ teaspoon dried tarragon
4 tablespoons of sun-dried tomato pesto
1 red pepper, sliced
400 ml chicken stock
600–800 ml water
1 × 400 g can of butter beans, drained (230 g dry weight)
Black pepper to season

Method

1. Heat half the oil in a large non-stick frying pan. Add the diced chicken to the pan and fry until cooked through. Remove the chicken from the pan and set aside.
2. Heat the remaining oil in the same frying pan and cook the diced onion for a few minutes without colouring until starting to soften.
3. Add the pearl barley, dried tarragon, pesto, red pepper and stock. Bring to the boil, then lower the heat so that it is just simmering. You will need to add some or all of the water as the pearl barley grains swell. Simmer for 45–60 minutes until the stock is absorbed and the barley is tender but still has a little bite. Return the chicken to the pan, add the butter beans, reheat, season with black pepper and serve.

Cooking Tip Cut down on cooking time by pre-cooking the pearl barley or replacing it with brown rice. You could experiment with other canned beans.

COD WITH LIME-CRUSHED NEW POTATOES

Preparation time: minimum 20 minutes
Cooking time: 20 minutes
Serves 4

Ingredients

Juice and zest of 1 small lemon
1 heaped teaspoon harissa paste
1 tablespoon honey
2 tablespoons chopped flat leaf parsley
4 × 150 g cod fillets
1 tablespoon extra virgin olive oil plus a little extra for
  greasing
600 g new potatoes, cleaned
Juice and zest of 1 lime
Vegetables of your choice, to serve

Method

1. Mix together the lemon juice and zest, harissa paste, honey and parsley in a shallow dish. Marinade the fish in the mixture for a minimum of 15 minutes and up to 2 hours.
2. Preheat the oven to 180°C with a metal baking tray inside.
3. Cut a piece of cooking foil big enough to parcel the fish in and brush lightly with extra virgin olive oil.
4. Put the fish and marinade into the foil and seal into a parcel.
5. Place the foil parcel on to the heated baking tray and cook the fish for 15–20 minutes or until just cooked.
6. Boil the potatoes for 15 minutes until just tender.
7. Coarsely mash the potatoes with a tablespoon of extra virgin olive oil and the zest and juice of the lime.
8. Serve with vegetables of your choice, such as lightly baked cherry tomatoes and steamed mangetout.

Cooking Tip If short for time, paint the harissa paste on to the cod and bake without the other marinade ingredients.

CREAMY FISH PIE

Preparation time: 30 minutes
Cooking time: 30 minutes
Serves 4

Ingredients

750 g floury potatoes such as Maris Piper, peeled and cut into
   pieces
1 tablespoon sunflower spread
2–3 tablespoons skimmed milk
2 leeks, finely sliced
1 tablespoon olive or rapeseed oil
200 g young spinach leaves
400 g smoked undyed haddock boned, skinned and cut into
   small pieces
120 g smoked salmon offcuts
100 g frozen peas, defrosted
75 g light crème fraîche
Black pepper to season

Method

1. Preheat the oven to 200°C.
2. Boil the potatoes until cooked. Drain, season and mash
   with the sunflower spread and a little milk. Leave to one
   side to cool.
3. While the potatoes cook, gently sweat the leeks in the olive
   oil in a pan with a lid over a low heat, taking care not to
   brown them. When soft, add the spinach and cook for a
   few minutes or so until it wilts.
4. Take half of the spinach and leek mixture, season and mix
   with the crème fraîche. Blend using a hand blender. It will
   make a bright green sauce.

5. Season the smoked haddock and arrange with the salmon and peas in a deep ovenproof dish. Pour the creamy green sauce over the fish and peas.
6. Carefully top with the remaining spinach and leek mixture and then the mashed potato. Smooth the potato then use a fork to make a circular pattern on the top.
7. Cook for 30 minutes, until the sauce is bubbling and the potato starting to brown.
8. Serve with one or two additional vegetables.

HUNTER CHICKEN

Preparation time: 10 minutes
Cooking time: 35–45 minutes
Serves 4

Ingredients

4 chicken legs or 8 chicken pieces, skin and fat removed
2 tablespoons olive oil
1 large onion, diced
1 clove of garlic, crushed or finely diced
2 celery sticks, finely diced
400 g can of chopped tomatoes
150 g diced mushrooms
2 tablespoons sun-dried tomato paste
1 bay leaf
1 teaspoon dried tarragon
250 mls white wine
200 mls chicken stock

Method

1. Brown the chicken in the oil in a frying pan. Set the chicken aside but keep warm.

2. In the same pan cook the onion and garlic for a few minutes without colouring. Add the celery and continue to cook for a further few minutes.
3. Blitz the chopped tomatoes to a purée using a hand blender (optional).
4. Return the chicken to the pan, with the tomatoes, mushrooms, tomato paste, herbs, wine and chicken stock.
5. Bring to the boil, reduce to a simmer and cover. Cook for 25–35 minutes, checking to see if the chicken is cooked all the way through.

Cooking Tip Great served with a starchy vegetable or wholegrain that soaks up the juices such as butter beans, potato and celeriac mash, polenta or couscous.

PAELLA

Preparation time: 10 minutes
Cooking time: 25 minutes
Serves 4

Ingredients

1 large onion, peeled and diced
1 clove garlic, crushed
1 teaspoon paprika
1–2 tablespoons olive oil
2 red peppers, diced
300 g Arborio rice
1 litre chicken or turkey stock
150 g cherry tomatoes
200 g diced cooked chicken or turkey (dark meat works well)
A handful of freshly chopped parsley
80 g defrosted peas

250–300 g frozen paella mix (shelled mussels, squid,
   prawns, etc.)
Salt (if needed) and pepper
1 lemon, quartered and visible pips removed

Method

1. Cook the onion, garlic and paprika gently in the oil in a
   large frying pan for a few minutes, taking care not to brown
   the onion.
2. When the onion starts to become translucent, add the diced
   peppers and then the rice, stirring for a couple of minutes
   in between. Continue to stir the rice mixture for two more
   minutes.
3. Add a couple of ladles of the stock to the mixture and the
   tomatoes. Turn down the heat until it is just simmering.
   The rice will take about 20 minutes to cook from now.
4. Continue to add the stock a ladle at a time, allowing the
   rice to absorb the stock. After 10 minutes add the diced
   cooked chicken or turkey. About 4 or 5 minutes from the
   end add the parsley, peas and the fish mixture and continue
   to cook.
5. Check the rice and fish are cooked before serving, season
   with salt and pepper to taste.
6. Serve with wedges of lemon.

Cooking Tip Great for using up leftover turkey or chicken –
especially the darker more flavoursome meat.

PORK AND PINEAPPLE

Preparation time: 10 minutes
Cooking time: 1 hour 10 minutes
Serves 4

Ingredients

2 tablespoons vegetable oil
1 large or 2 small onions, chopped
400 g pork steak cut into pieces
½–1 teaspoon garam masala
½–1 teaspoon ground cinnamon
½–1 teaspoon chilli powder
½–1 teaspoon ground ginger
1 × 400 g can of chopped tomatoes in their juices
150 ml water
110 g pineapple slices cut into chunks (with their juices)
1 × 410 g can of green lentils

Method

1. Preheat the oven to 180°C.
2. Heat 1 tablespoon of the oil and fry the onion without colour until softened.
3. Add the pork and brown on all sides.
4. Transfer the pork and onion to an ovenproof dish and add all the other ingredients. Stir to mix.
5. Cook in the oven for about an hour or until tender.
6. Serve with one or more vegetables of your choice.

SMOKED SALMON FISH CAKES

Preparation time: 20 minutes
Cooking time: 20 minutes
Serves 4–5 (makes 8–10)

Ingredients

500 g floury potatoes, such as Maris Piper or Vivaldi, peeled and boiled

200 g smoked salmon pieces or trimmings
2 tablespoons chopped chives
Zest of one lemon
4 spring onions, finely chopped (use both the green and the white parts)
1 tablespoon extra virgin olive oil
Black pepper
50 g plain flour
2 eggs, beaten
100 g wholemeal breadcrumbs

Method

1. Preheat the oven to 220°C.
2. Cook the potatoes in boiling water for around 20 minutes or until tender. Drain, mash and allow to cool.
3. Add the smoked salmon pieces, chopped chives, lemon zest, spring onions and olive oil to the cooled potato.
4. Season with black pepper and mix together. Scoop up 3–4 tablespoons of the mixture and use your hands to form into patties.
5. Spread the flour on to a plate. Dip all the patties in the flour so they are covered all over in a thin layer. Then dip each one in the beaten egg followed by breadcrumbs.
6. Assemble on a non-stick baking sheet and bake for 20 minutes.
7. Serve with green salad and sweet chilli sauce.

Cooking Tip These fish cakes can be made the day before, stored in the fridge and cooked when needed. Alternatively make them in bulk and freeze. You will need to increase the cooking time by 10 minutes if cooking from frozen.

QUICK STIR FRY

Preparation time: 10–15 minutes
Cooking time: 20 minutes
Serves 2

Ingredients

Selection of easy-cook vegetables such as peas, edamame beans, sweetcorn, thinly sliced courgettes, fine beans, thinly sliced carrots, peppers (about 150–250 g in weight)
65 g egg noodles
1 small onion, sliced
1 large or 2 small cloves garlic, crushed
1 tablespoon rapeseed or toasted sesame oil
100–140 g leftover meat such as pork or chicken, or use quorn or firm tofu pieces
3–4 tablespoons chicken or vegetable stock
2 tablespoons light soy sauce
2 tablespoons rice wine vinegar
2 teaspoons sugar
½ inch finely grated ginger (about 1 teaspoon)
1 teaspoon Chinese five-spice powder
2 teaspoons cornflour mixed well with a little water

Method

1. You will need to cook any starchy vegetables (carrots, broccoli, fine beans) in boiling water for a few minutes until almost tender but still firm.
2. Cook the noodles in boiling water for a few minutes or as per the packet instructions.
3. Cook the sliced onion and garlic in the oil in a wok or non-stick frying pan for 3–4 minutes, taking care not to brown it.

4. Add the drained vegetables together with any peas, sweet-corn, peppers, defrosted edamame beans, courgette strips to the pan and continue to stir fry.

5. Shred or cut any meat you are using into fine slices, add this or the quorn or tofu pieces to the wok or frying pan at this stage, stir for a few minutes to warm through.

6. Add the stock, soy sauce, vinegar, sugar, ginger, five-spice powder, and lastly the cornflour mix to the pan and stir immediately. Continue to cook for about a minute until the sauce thickens.

7. Serve in warmed bowls on top of the drained noodles.

SPICED NUT AND VEGGIE BURGERS

Preparation time: 10–15 minutes
Cooking time: 20 minutes
Makes 8–10 burgers

Ingredients

1 onion, finely chopped
1 garlic clove, crushed
2 tablespoons rapeseed oil
125 g mixed nuts
1 tablespoons harissa paste
Zest of one lemon
Large handful fresh coriander leaves
Juice of half a lemon
1 × 400 g can of kidney beans drained
1 × 400 g can of sweetcorn
4 burger buns
Salad and chutney, to serve

Method

1. Cook the onion and garlic in half the oil until soft, but not browned. Allow to cool.
2. Place the onion mixture, mixed nuts, harissa paste, lemon zest, fresh coriander, lemon juice and half the kidney beans in a food processor and pulse until you have a coarse paste.
3. Add the remaining kidney beans and the sweetcorn and lightly pulse so that there are still pieces of the kidney beans and sweetcorn visible.
4. Remove from the processor, divide the mixture into 8 equal-sized portions (about 100 g each) and form into burger shapes.
5. Cover your grill pan tray with foil and lightly oil. Place the burgers on top and brush with a little oil.
6. Grill under a medium heat for around 20 minutes, turning every 5 minutes and brushing with oil if needed. The burgers may tend to split so turn them carefully.
7. Toast the burger buns. Serve the burgers on top of the buns with your favourite salad topping and chutney.

Cooking Tip You can prepare the burgers up to 24 hours in advance. Keep them covered in the fridge and cook them when you need them. Alternatively, store them in the freezer. You can cook from frozen but increase the cooking time by about 10 minutes.

NUT LOAF

Preparation time: 40 minutes
Cooking time: 1 hour
Serves 8

Ingredients

2 aubergines
3–4 tablespoons olive oil
1 medium onion, finely chopped
2 stalks of celery, finely chopped
2 cloves garlic, crushed
200 g mixed nuts (such as almonds, Brazil nuts, cashews,
    hazelnuts, pecans, pine nuts, pistachio, walnuts)
110 g wholemeal breadcrumbs
1 teaspoon dried oregano
2 tablespoons chopped fresh coriander leaves
Zest and juice from 1 lemon
2 eggs
100 g grated low-fat Cheddar cheese
Salt and pepper

Method

1. Preheat the oven to 180°C.
2. Thinly slice the aubergines lengthwise. Brush both sides
   with olive oil and season. Cook under a medium grill for a
   few minutes, then turn, brush with oil and repeat. The
   aubergine should start to soften and colour.
3. Oil a 2-pound loaf tin and use the cooled aubergines to line
   the tin. Make sure all the slices are going in the same direc-
   tion and leave sufficient aubergine to top the filling.
4. Cook the onion, celery and garlic in 1 tablespoon of olive
   oil, taking care not to colour the onion.
5. Chop the nuts in a food processor, but not too finely. Place
   these together with the breadcrumbs, herbs, lemon zest,
   beaten egg, grated cheese, cooked onion and celery in a
   bowl, season and mix. Add about half the lemon juice.
6. Place the nut mixture into the loaf tin, making sure that it
   is pressed into all the corners and flattened down. Cover
   with the remaining aubergine.

7. Protect the top of the loaf with foil to prevent burning and roast in the oven for an hour.
8. Allow to cool for a few minutes. Place a serving plate over the loaf and flip over. If all goes well you should be able to turn the loaf out ready for slicing and serving.
9. Serve while warm with vegetables of your choice and a helping of the rich tomato sauce on page 239. It can also be enjoyed cold with salad or for packed lunches.

Sides

ROASTED AUBERGINE AND BABA GANOUSH

Preparation time: 10 minutes
Cooking time: 25 minutes
Serves 8 as a vegetable and 16–20 as a dip

Ingredients for the roasted aubergine

4 large aubergines
4 cloves of garlic, sliced
1½ tablespoons extra virgin oil
Salt and pepper

Additional ingredients for the baba ganoush

100 g sesame seeds
1 teaspoon paprika
Juice of 1 lemon
1½ tablespoons extra virgin oil if needed
Salt and pepper
Coriander or parsley, to garnish

Method – to serve as a vegetable

1. Preheat the oven to 200°C.
2. Cut the aubergines in half lengthways. Make some slits in the flesh with a sharp knife and poke in pieces of the garlic clove. You might need to use your knife to prise open the slits a little. Brush generously with oil and season with a little salt and pepper. Roast flesh side up for around 40–45 minutes. Check about halfway through cooking and if necessary cover with foil to prevent them from burning.

Method – to serve as a dip

1. Roast the aubergines as above.
2. Place the sesame seeds in a heavy frying pan and toast over a high heat for a few minutes, stirring constantly until lightly toasted. Take care not to burn them. Transfer the seeds to a dish and allow to cool. Once cool, blitz in a coffee grinder or grind with a pestle and mortar to a fine paste.
3. When the aubergines are cool enough to handle, scoop out the flesh into a blender, add the sesame seed powder, paprika and lemon juice and blitz to a purée (or use a bowl and hand blender). Add the remaining oil as necessary to achieve the right consistency for a dip and season to taste.
4. Tip into a serving bowl, garnish with parsley or coriander and serve with strips of toasted wholemeal pitta bread.
5. Freeze any of the dip you don't need for another time.

EDAMAME BEAN DIP

Preparation time: 10 minutes
Cooking time: 2–3 minutes
Serves 8

Ingredients

80 g frozen edamame beans, thawed
50 g frozen peas, thawed
50 g canned cannellini beans
1½ tablespoons mint sauce
1½ tablespoons lemon juice
1 clove garlic
1 tablespoon extra virgin oil
3 tablespoons light crème fraîche
Pinch salt, if needed
Black pepper

Method

1. Cook the edamame beans and peas until tender.
2. Place the edamame beans, peas, cannellini beans, mint sauce, lemon juice, garlic clove and olive oil in a food processor and blitz to a fine paste.
3. Mix in the crème fraîche to your desired consistency and season to taste.
4. Serve with sticks of carrot, celery, cucumber and peppers.

SMOKED MACKEREL PÂTÉ

Preparation time: 5 minutes
Serves 4

Ingredients

225 g smoked mackerel fillets
6 tablespoons light crème fraîche
Juice of half a lemon
Black pepper
1 tablespoon of horseradish sauce (optional)

Method

1. Remove the skin from the mackerel and remove any bones.
2. Place the flesh in a food processor with the other ingredients.
3. Blend until smooth and season to taste.
4. Chill until ready to serve. Goes well with toasted wholegrain or multigrain bread.

SPICY STIR-FRIED OKRA

Preparation time: 10 minutes
Cooking time: 10–12 minutes
Serves 4

Ingredients

500 g okra
1 tablespoon olive oil
1 teaspoon cumin seeds
2 large onions, thickly sliced
1 green chilli, deseeded and finely chopped
¼ teaspoon ground turmeric
½ teaspoon red chilli powder
½ teaspoon salt
½ teaspoon garam masala
1 tablespoon freshly chopped coriander leaf

Method

1. Trim the heads and tails of the okra, then cut into 5 cm-long pieces. Slit each horizontally without cutting into two.
2. Heat the oil in a non-stick wok and add the cumin seeds. Sauté briefly, then add the onions and green chilli and cook for 2–3 minutes.

3. Add the okra, then sprinkle on the turmeric, chilli powder and salt. Mix well, cover, and cook over a low heat for 5 minutes, stirring occasionally. Add the garam masala and cook for a further 2 minutes. Add the freshly chopped coriander, stir briefly and serve.

Cooking Tip Okra, or lady's fingers, cooked in this simple manner are delicious in a wrap or with noodles.

TOMATO SAUCE

Preparation time: 5 minutes
Cooking time: 30 minutes
Serves 4

Ingredients

1 large onion, finely diced
3 cloves of garlic, crushed
2 tablespoons olive oil
3 × 400 g cans chopped tomatoes
4 tablespoons of sun-dried tomato paste
A teaspoon of dried basil or oregano leaves
Black pepper to season
2 teaspoons balsamic vinegar

Method

1. Cook the garlic and onion in the oil, taking care not to colour the onion. This should take about 5 minutes.
2. Add the tomatoes, tomato paste and herbs to the pan; bring to a slow simmer and cook for a further 10–20 minutes.
3. Season with pepper and balsamic vinegar. If desired you can use a hand blender to liquidise the final sauce.

4. You can thicken the sauce more if required by adding a little flour and water and cooking for a few additional minutes or by adding more tomato paste.

Cooking Tip You can use this versatile sauce with the nut loaf on page 233, add it to pasta for a quick lunch or spread it on a pizza base.

Desserts and bakes

CHOCOLATE CAKE

Preparation time: 20 minutes
Cooking time: up to 2½ hours
Serves 12+

Ingredients

200 g beetroot
200 g soft brown sugar
100 ml sunflower oil
4 eggs, beaten
50 g plain low-fat yoghurt
Grated zest of 2 oranges
100 g dark chocolate (at least 70 per cent cocoa solids), melted
100 g wholemeal flour
100 g self-raising flour
2 teaspoons baking powder

Method

1. Prepare the beetroot by peeling, cutting into pieces and boiling for about 15–20 minutes until tender. Mash and leave to cool.

2. Preheat the oven to 190°C/170°C fan.
3. Grease and line a 20 cm (8 inch) round deep-sided cake tin.
4. Sieve the sugar into a large mixing bowl to ensure there are no lumps in it. Add the oil, eggs, yoghurt, orange zest, melted chocolate and mix.
5. Sift the two flours and baking powder into the mixture and fold in.
6. Add the beetroot purée and stir to mix.
7. Empty the mixture into the cake tin.
8. Place on a baking sheet in the oven and cook for 1½–2 hours or until a skewer comes out clean.
9. Leave to cool for a few minutes before turning out.

Fillings (optional)

You can leave the cake whole but could also split it in half horizontally and fill with:
Cherry or raspberry jam
Cherry or raspberry jam and reduced-fat whipped cream
Butter cream made from icing sugar and unsaturated 60 per cent fat spread. Keep the cake in the fridge between uses.

Topping (optional)

Top with melted dark chocolate (70 per cent cocoa solids) or with chocolate icing made from cocoa powder, icing sugar and a little orange juice.

CHOCOLATE SYRUP PUDDING

Preparation time: 10 minutes
Cooking time: 20 minutes
Serves 4

Ingredients

5 tablespoons cocoa powder
125 g soft brown sugar
200 mls hot water
80 g sunflower spread (use a 60% fat spread)
75 g self-raising flour
1 teaspoon baking powder
3 eggs

Method

1. Preheat the oven to 180°C.
2. In a bowl, mix together 2 tablespoons of the cocoa powder and 50 g of the sugar. Add a small amount of the hot water to form a paste. Mix until smooth, then slowly add the remaining hot water, ensuring there are no lumps. Set to one side.
3. Grease an ovenproof pudding dish with a little of the spread.
4. Pass the remaining cocoa, the flour and baking powder through a sieve.
5. Cream the remaining spread and sugar together, add each egg one at a time together with about a third of the flour mix. Beat well between each addition.
6. Put the chocolate pudding mix into the bottom of the greased pudding dish.
7. Stir the sauce mixture again and then carefully pour it over the pudding mix so that it sits on top.
8. Pop in the oven and bake for around 20 minutes.
9. When you remove from the oven you will have a light sponge with a lovely chocolate sauce beneath. It is nice served on its own or you could add a scoop of ice cream, dollop of soya or oat cream alternative, or a spoon or two of low-fat custard.

HEALTHY CRUMBLE MIXTURE

Preparation time: 15 minutes
Cooking time: 35–40 minutes
Serves 6

Ingredients

4 tablespoons honey
60 g sunflower spread (60% fat)
150 g rolled oats
50 g chopped almonds and hazelnuts
25 g pumpkin seeds
2 tablespoons oat bran
1 teaspoon ground cinnamon or mixed spice

Method

1. Preheat the oven to 180°C.
2. Warm the honey and sunflower spread together in a pan and stir to mix.
3. Assemble the oats and other dry ingredients together in a bowl.
4. Add the oat mixture to the pan and stir until thoroughly combined.
5. Place the fruit (see page 205 for stewed fruit recipe) in an ovenproof dish and top with the crumble mixture, taking care to spread evenly. Firm down the topping.
6. Bake for 35–40 minutes or until the crumble is golden brown.
7. Serve with low-fat custard, soy-cream alternative, low-fat yoghurt, non-dairy ice cream or low-fat crème fraîche.

Cooking Tip If you want a crispy crumble, make sure the stewed fruit is not too wet.

STICKY SWEET POTATO AND GINGER MARMALADE LOAF

Preparation time: 15 minutes
Cooking time: 1 hour 15 minutes
Makes 10–12 slices

Ingredients

2 eggs
150 ml vegetable oil
175 g light muscovado sugar, sieved
350 g sweet potatoes, peeled and finely grated
4 tablespoons thick-cut marmalade
1 tablespoon stem ginger, washed and chopped
200 g self-raising wholemeal flour
½ teaspoon bicarbonate of soda
1 teaspoon mixed spice
2 tablespoons orange juice

Method

1. Preheat the oven to 150°C. Grease and line a 2 lb loaf tin.
2. Beat the eggs with the oil and sugar. Stir in the sweet potato, 2 tablespoons of the marmalade and the ginger pieces.
3. Sieve the flour, bicarbonate and mixed spice (together) into the egg, oil and sugar mixture, adding in any bran that is left in the sieve. Stir well to combine.
4. Pour into the lined tin, shake to level the surface and bake for 1 hour 15 minutes or until a skewer comes out clean.
5. Allow to cool in the tin then turn out on to a wire rack.
6. Heat the remaining marmalade and the orange juice together in a pan. Allow to cool slightly. Make holes in the top of the loaf and brush the mixture over the top.

BERRY AND ELDERFLOWER BOMB

Preparation time: 10 minutes
Setting time: 2–6 hours
Serves 8

Ingredients

500–550 g small (fresh) berry fruits such as small strawberries,
  raspberries, blackberries, redcurrants
4 gelatine leaves
450 ml cranberry juice or elderflower cordial diluted 1:4 with
  water
50 g caster sugar
2 pint round pudding bowl

Method

1. Wash and dry the fruit and mix together. Place in the
   pudding bowl.
2. Soak the gelatine leaves in cold water for 5 minutes.
3. Gently heat half the cordial or cranberry juice with the
   sugar in a saucepan. When it's almost boiling, remove any
   excess moisture from the gelatine leaves and add them to
   the pan. Stir occasionally until melted. Don't allow the
   mixture to boil.
4. Pour the mixture back into the jug and top up with the
   remaining juice or cordial, mix and leave to cool.
5. Once cooled, pour about two-thirds of the mixture over the
   fruit. You now need to weigh this down while it sets. To do
   this, cover loosely with cling film and then weigh down
   with a small saucer with a heavy weight on top, something
   like a can of beans or a jar of jam. Transfer to the fridge for
   a couple of hours.

6. Once firm, remove the weight, add the remaining jelly mix and leave to set. If the remaining jelly has already set you may need to warm it gently in a pan or in a microwave.

7. To turn out, dip the bowl in a pan of hot water until the jelly just starts to melt, top with a plate, turn upside down and hold your breath. Return to the fridge until needed. Slice with a sharp knife and serve with a low-fat pouring cream, low-fat yoghurt mixed with a little honey, or with half-fat crème fraîche.

Cooking Tip You can replace the cordial or cranberry juice with a sparkling wine for a special occasion.

CARROT AND PINEAPPLE MUFFINS

Preparation time: 15–20 minutes
Cooking time: 40 minutes
Makes 12 muffins

Ingredients

200 g carrots, cooked then mashed
85 g wholemeal flour
2 teaspoons ground cinnamon
½ teaspoon bicarbonate of soda
150 ml sunflower oil
100 g caster sugar
140 g self-raising flour
140 g pineapple (canned or fresh), cut into small chunks
2 tablespoons pineapple juice
50 g sunflower seeds
1 large egg
1 teaspoon vanilla extract

Method

1. Pre-cook the carrot in boiling water, drain, mash and leave to cool.
2. Preheat the oven to 200°C.
3. Sift the flours, cinnamon and bicarbonate of soda together into a bowl.
4. In another bowl beat together the sunflower oil and the sugar.
5. Add the cooled mashed carrot, pineapple chunks, pineapple juice, sunflower seeds, egg and vanilla extract to the oil and sugar and mix.
6. Fold in the dry ingredients.
7. Spoon the mixture into muffin, cupcake or bun cases and bake for 20 minutes.

BREAD AND BUTTER SURPRISE PUDDING

Preparation time: 10 minutes
Cooking time: 25–30 minutes
Serves 4

Ingredients

6 teaspoons 60% sunflower spread
6 slices of wholemeal bread or a 50:50 bread
50 g ready-to-eat apricots, chopped
50 g caster sugar
2 eggs
250 mls reduced-fat single cream, or better still use a soya or oat cream alternative
1 teaspoon vanilla extract
1 teaspoon soft brown sugar
50 g chopped dark chocolate

Method

1. Grease the inside of a casserole dish with the sunflower spread.
2. Cut the crusts from the bread and spread with the remaining sunflower spread. Cut each slice into quarters.
3. You need to arrange the bread in layers in the casserole dish. Start by putting in a layer of bread, spread side up, in the dish. Sprinkle over about one third of the apricots and chopped chocolate. Repeat with two more layers of bread, fruit and chocolate and then the final layer of bread, spread side down.
4. Beat the eggs with the caster sugar, then add the cream and the vanilla essence.
5. Pour over the pudding and leave to stand. This allows the bread to soak up all the juices from the custardy sauce. Sprinkle the soft brown sugar on top.
6. Preheat the oven to 180°C.
7. After 30 minutes of standing the pudding should be ready for the oven. Bake for 25–30 minutes.
8. It should come out hot, golden and crisp. Serve on its own or with a little low-fat cream, or light crème fraîche.

Cooking Tip You can prepare ahead of time and keep in the fridge until you need to cook it.

Case studies

I
t is surprising how much we learn by listening to other people's stories. It brings the problem of dealing with high cholesterol to life and above all emphasises that you are not alone in dealing with the issue. Maybe you can see yourself in one of these stories? They are all based on real-life case studies but some of the details, including names, have been changed.

Of course everyone is unique and it is unlikely that your medical history and background will be identical to any of the cases featured below. This book and these case studies can only offer you guidance. It is important, if you are worried about your health and/or your treatment, that you speak to your doctor, dietitian or nurse to find out what is the best course of action for you.

Case study 1 – Exercise

David, a 55-year-old accountant on statins, is looking to become more active but he is worried about whether this might aggravate a pre-existing knee problem. He chats with his doctor who refers him to the local gym for advice. At the gym a trained instructor advises him and gives him an initial programme of activity. As David progresses and becomes more confident the exercise is built up week by week. David learns that physical activity can help him avoid a range of health conditions as well as improve his cholesterol readings. When he returns to the clinic months later he tells his GP that he is now wearing trousers two sizes smaller, has lost a little weight, strengthened his knee and is generally feeling very positive. His GP is delighted, especially as his HDL cholesterol (good cholesterol) has increased and his blood pressure seems better. Here is the advice that the fitness instructor gave David.

- Start slowly and gradually build exercise up to 150+ minutes every week
- Change a few daily habits (e.g. avoid sitting down for long periods, try walking more each day)
- Choose activities you enjoy
- Don't exercise if you feel unwell or if your knee is playing up
- Stop the activity or exercise if you're in pain or feel dizzy, don't overdo it
- Avoid exercise within two hours of a main meal. The output from your heart rises by 20 per cent to cope with digestion, so exercising too soon could make you feel unwell
- Wear comfortable shoes and clothes
- Start slowly to warm up and build up the pace of your activity gradually. Make sure you slow down gradually too.
- Remember to drink water before, during and after your activity
- Do some stretching exercises before and after your activity to help avoid muscle stiffness or strain the next day.

For more details on exercise see chapter 8.

Case study 2 – Dietary improvements

Jean, a 49-year-old admin clerk, has always thought of herself as very healthy. So it comes as a bit of a shock when her recent blood results reveal her total cholesterol is 6.2, HDL 1.7 and LDL 3.9 mmol/l. Although her GP is not concerned, Jean is worried.

Jean's total cholesterol and LDL are above 5 and 3 so ideally it would be good to bring these down. Happily Jean's HDL is at a healthy level. Her GP explains that cholesterol is only one risk factor out of many and asks about other risk factors.

Jean's GP inputs all Jean's relevant medical history into a cardiovascular risk calculator and assesses her risk of a heart attack or stroke over the next 10 years as low, so is not overly concerned with her cholesterol results. However, her GP still recommends that Jean might benefit from trying to reduce her cholesterol levels further by improving her diet and lifestyle. He provides her with some general guidance and suggests she visit the HEART UK website for more information. Jean tweeks her diet to include cholesterol-lowering foods and increases her physical activity. She was delighted to find that her blood test results after three months of following the revised diet and lifestyle showed that her lipid levels were all vastly improved.

Case study 3 – Possible FH

Angela, who is 40, was told her cholesterol was 7.8 mmol/l following an NHS health check and was too high. She was not given her LDL or HDL cholesterol results.

Ideally total cholesterol should be below 5 mmol/l, LDL cholesterol below 3 mmol/l and HDL above 1.2 mmol/l, but it is generally accepted by most lipid experts that the lower the total and LDL cholesterol the better. In people with diabetes, high blood pressure, existing heart problems or those with a family history of heart disease, the total cholesterol and LDL should be lower than this.

Latest guidance suggests that individual targets should be set for each person ideally reducing LDL cholesterol by 40 per cent from baseline. However a total cholesterol over 7.5 or an LDL cholesterol above 4.9 is suggestive of a condition called

FH (see chapter 3, page 29) familial hypercholesterolemia which is an inherited condition.

Angela's GP asks Angela if she is aware of any premature heart disease in either side of her family as this might help with a diagnosis. Angela was separated from her father at a young age but thinks he died early of a heart attack. Angela's doctor thinks it is possible that Angela may have FH so refers her to a lipid clinic where a formal diagnosis can be made. This involves a fasting blood test, a physical examination and taking more details about her family's history of heart disease. It may even involve doing a genetic test. At the clinic the specialist completes a pedigree – a family tree to help identify any pattern of family members affected by inherited high cholesterol or early heart disease. As a result of all the investigations the doctor thinks that it is unlikely that Angela has FH, but because her cholesterol is significantly raised he arranges for her to see a dietitian and come back in three months.

It is important to get a diagnosis of FH early because, with effective treatment, people with FH can live a full and healthy life. If Angela did have FH the specialist would talk to her about contacting other family members that might also be affected. If Angela has any children, they would be invited for screening too. Children of people affected by FH should ideally be screened before they are 10 years old but not before the age of 2 years.

Case Study 4 – Statins

Muriel, an active 71-year-old, was recently told by her GP that she has a 23 per cent risk of a heart attack in the next 10 years and was advised to take a statin. However Muriel is adamant that she doesn't want to take any kind of tablet.

Muriel is at high risk of a heart attack or stroke. She is well within her rights to refuse to take a statin but she should be fully informed before she makes the decision not to accept treatment. It is recommended that GPs offer to prescribe a statin for people who have a 10 per cent (1 in 10) or greater risk of having a heart attack or stroke in the next 10 years. It is possible that if Muriel has a stroke or a heart attack it may be fatal or it might result in significant disability, something Muriel might find difficult given her active lifestyle.

Muriel decides not to take a statin, after listening to the advice from her doctor, but wants to maximise the changes she can make to her lifestyle. Her doctor agrees a three-month trial to see if Muriel can reduce her cholesterol levels and recommends that she discusses her options again with him once the trial period is over.

Increasing age accounts for a large proportion of the risk of having a heart attack or stroke. So as she gets older, Muriel's risk will only increase. All adults over 75 are generally considered at high risk. Despite negative media to the contrary, millions of people take statins safely and effectively and they are usually well tolerated by most!

After a three-month trial period, and with Muriel following the 4 Steps, her cholesterol results were improved, but her doctor still advised taking statins. Having read up on statins, Muriel agreed, but still sticks to her new healthier lifestyle whilst also taking medication.

Case study 5 – Low HDL, high triglycerides

Mark, a 50-year-old IT engineer, was recently diagnosed with raised cholesterol which he has managed to control. However his HDL (good cholesterol) remains low (0.6 mmol/l) and his triglycerides (TG) are still raised.

A raised TG level and a reduced HDL often go hand in hand and are two of the key features of metabolic syndrome, a well-known collection of symptoms that increases the risk of cardiovascular disease and diabetes. Reduced HDL cholesterol and increased TGs are also symptoms of familial combined hyperlipidaemia (FCH), an inherited condition which affects 1 in 100 people.

Mark's doctor advises him that HDL-cholesterol levels in men should ideally be above 1.0 mmol/l and that HDL levels above 1.5 mmol/l may give even greater protection against vascular disease. She advises him that there are some things that he can do to increase his HDL levels although this will take some effort on his part. By the time Mark leaves the surgery he understands that if he continues to gain weight, smoke and eat badly then his chances of having a heart attack and developing diabetes before he plans to retire at 60 are high. However stopping smoking, moderate weight loss, reducing any fat around his waistline, improving his diet and increasing activity can all help to improve his health.

Mark is trying to follow this advice and has been given lots of support and encouragement to help him stop smoking. He is also trying to cut the cravings by using nicotine patches. He has seen an increase in his appetite, so he is trying to prevent weight gain by doing more exercise using an app on his phone that measures the number of steps he takes each day. He has already increased his steps from 2000 to 5000 on most days. Now three months later Mark has had a recent blood test and is waiting for his next appointment to see the results. He couldn't wait to find out if he had already made a difference so he asked the receptionist, who confirmed that his HDL was now 1.1 mmol/l.

Mark has also been online to find out about what else he can do to help himself. He learnt that any exercise he does should be of at least moderate intensity and frequency (see chapter 8 on exercise) and last for at least 30 minutes each day. In terms of dietary changes, he now knows that adopting a very low-fat diet is not the best approach as it may reduce his HDL levels further. In the long term he is aiming to lose some weight around his waistline, by limiting his sweet tooth, cutting down on portion sizes and reducing his alcohol intake.

He also knows that two to four portions of oily fish each week are recommended for men and post-menopausal women with raised triglycerides. He is not a fan of fish so for the moment this is on hold. His wife is delighted to see the change in his appearance and energy levels.

Case Study 6 – A heart attack story

Michael, a 65-year-old retired mechanic, had his cholesterol levels checked at a local pharmacy two weeks after his first heart attack. It had gone right down despite him not having taken the statin his doctor prescribed. Michael was delighted, but his cardiologist did not seem as pleased as Michael was.

Dr Babar explained that after a heart attack, cholesterol levels usually fall, but they return to the usual level after two to three months. Michael later explained to his wife that cholesterol measurements taken 24 hours after a heart attack and up to three months later are considered unreliable because they tend to be low and therefore falsely reassuring. Michael's enthusiasm was initially checked but he decided to sign up for the cardiac rehabilitation classes that his cardiologist recommended. Now a few months later he is on the mend, regularly taking a statin, and learning to take life a little easier. He always loved swimming and is planning to take it up again now he has retired as well as get involved in some local community activities. At a routine check-up his GP was happy with his progress and advised him that he would be calling him regularly for check-ups in the future.

Case Study 7 – Feeling run down on a statin

Vicky, a type 2 diabetic aged 55, has been taking rosuvastatin for over a year. Lately she has been feeling run down and decided to take a high-dose multivitamin and mineral supplement and a 'pick-me-up' tonic. She came across an article that seemed to indicate that if you are taking nicotinic acid (which is related to niacin, also known as vitamin B3) and a statin, this could increase the likelihood of muscle damage.

Vicky rang the HEART UK Cholesterol Helpline and was advised that she did not need to worry because the form of niacin in a general multivitamin and mineral tablet is safe to take with a statin. Nicotinic acid is only ever found in medicines and in recent years these have been withdrawn in the UK. She was also advised that when opting for a vitamin and mineral supplement up to 100 per cent of the Labelling Reference Intake (RI) should not cause a problem with any statin, including rosuvastatin (see page 133). She spoke to a very helpful dietitian who explained that this is roughly the amount that we should all be taking in as part of a healthy diet. Some supplements, she was told, do contain much higher levels of vitamins and minerals and Vicky should take care with these especially as she is also taking a tonic as well as the supplement. Vicky learnt that it was only too easy to exceed the recommended intake of some nutrients such as vitamin A (retinol) and iron by taking one or more supplements at the same time. If, after taking a supplement for a couple of weeks, she feels little or no benefit in spite of a healthy balanced diet, Vicky was advised that she should discontinue the supplement(s) and check with her GP. Something other than her diet may be causing her to feel run down.

Case Study 8 – Starting a family

Lisa, now 24, was diagnosed with familial hypercholesterolaemia (FH) in her teens and has been on statins ever since. Now married, Lisa is planning to start a family and is concerned about the effect her statin may have on the unborn baby and if her children will inherit the condition.

Dr Griffin, who runs a family clinic for people with FH at Lisa's local hospital, advised that, as with all medications, it is difficult to know exactly what effect statins might have on an unborn baby. After a long discussion with the doctor Lisa agreed with her partner that she should follow the doctor's advice to stop her statin and her oral contraceptive at least three months before she plans to conceive and to take other precautions to prevent getting pregnant during that period. Lisa was also surprised that the doctor questioned her husband about his family's health and any history of raised cholesterol or early heart disease. He explained that there was a 1 in 2 chance of Lisa giving birth to a baby who might inherit the same FH-causing gene, but that he wanted some reassurance that her partner did not also have FH which would increase the risk for the baby. Fortunately Anthony, Lisa's partner, has recently had a cholesterol test at work and was advised this was normal.

The leaflet that Dr Griffin gave Lisa explained that a 3-month period allows for the statin to be used up by the body, so none is present in her blood when she falls pregnant. It also explained that Lisa should stay off her statin while she is pregnant and also while she is breastfeeding. If she chooses not to breastfeed, she can start her statin again once her baby is born.

Lisa now understands that FH is a genetically inherited disorder which is autosomally dominant. This means that each child born to Lisa and Anthony has a 50:50 (1 in 2) chance of inheriting FH. However if Anthony also had FH the chances of a baby being affected by FH increase to 75:25 (3 in 4) and it is possible that 1 in 4 children would be very severely affected. To be absolutely sure Anthony plans to get his cholesterol checked again by his GP before Lisa conceives, and check with his mum if there is any history of premature heart disease or high cholesterol in his family.

Case Study 9 – What's good for Dad works for the rest of the family

Philip, a long-term smoker, went for a routine blood test and was told he had high cholesterol. His GP gave him three months to try a diet and lifestyle approach to reducing his cholesterol. After three months his blood test was repeated to see what difference he had made and if he needed to start medication.

Initially Philip was not sure where to start as he has never had to worry about his weight, always being slightly under-weight, and consequently he normally ate whatever he fancied.

Unfortunately there was little support at the busy GP surgery to help Philip identify what he needed to do next. However, with help from his wife, a little research on the Internet and the advice of a family friend, he was able to make some headway. Philip's plan was to improve his cholesterol by:

- Stopping smoking. He learnt that about 20 per cent of heart disease deaths are directly attributable to smoking. (see page 27). Fortunately help was available when Philip signed up online on the NHS Smoke Free website. They sent him a free stop smoking kit and he was able to download a free stop smoking app and receive regular emails and texts to his phone to help and encourage him. It's not been easy, but so far Philip has cut his cigarettes right down to 5 a day and his plan is to stop completely within the next few weeks.

- Eating a healthier diet. Rebecca, Philip's wife, has been changing the way the whole family eat and they all feel better for it, including his two teenage sons. They love travelling to their holiday home in Italy and so have adopted a more Mediterranean way of eating. Rebecca has been building up a small repertoire of easy-to-cook dishes including a Mediterrean fish stew, Basil Chicken with Vermicelli and a favourite Bean Cassoulet. Rebecca now understands that she needs to replace animal fats like butter and lard with healthier oils and spreads, cut down on dairy fats and use smaller and leaner cuts of meat. More fresh vegetables, fruit and nuts are also regulars on the shopping list.

• Being physically active. Now he is smoking less Philip has started to go for a regular walk around the block every day for 30 minutes.

At his follow-up appointment Philip's GP was very pleased with him and decided that Philip did not need any medication at this stage. All the family were delighted and plans are afoot to celebrate with a self-catering activity weekend break.

Summary

All of our case studies made the decision to put diet and life-style change at the centre of their efforts to reduce their cholesterol. They understood from the start that it would not be easy to change habits that had, over the years, become ingrained in their daily routines. If they could speak to us now they would probably put their success down to four things:

1. Lots of support obtained from a variety of sources including friends, family, health professionals, heart charities and employers.
2. Planning – by making a plan and trying their very best to stick to it, they were ready for most eventualities.
3. Understanding the reasons for and wanting to make a change for the better to improve their physical and mental health and well-being
4. Making small changes and building these up over time rather than trying to do too much and failing at the first hurdle.

We hope you have enjoyed reading these stories and can build your own success too.

Frequently asked questions

How often do you have a burning question that you just can't find an answer to? It can be extremely frustrating when you can't find the right person to ask, or you get different opinions and don't know which one is right. On the HEART UK Cholesterol Helpline we have lots of experience of the niggling questions people want answers to. Here are a few of the most commonly asked, but if you have a burning question that is not covered here – check out the HEART UK website or call or email HEART UK's Cholesterol Helpline.

Q. Which is the best oil to use for cooking?

A. Any oils that you use should contain high amounts of mono- and polyunsaturated fats with minimal saturated fats. Different fats and oils have different uses. Each performs best within a certain range of temperatures. Some are better for high heat cooking, while others have intense flavours that are best enjoyed drizzled on salads.

Heating oil can change its characteristics. Some oils that are healthy at room temperature can become unhealthy when heated above certain temperatures.

When choosing cooking oil it is important to consider its smoking point. This is the temperature at which the fat begins to smoke and smell. The higher the smoking point, the better it performs at high temperatures. Processing, re-use, age and improper storage can all lower the smoking point. When oil smokes, it loses some of its health-promoting properties, so for the healthiest approach discard any oil that has gone beyond its smoke point.

Unsaturated oils become more saturated as you cook with them. For example, the oil in which we fry chips will become more saturated over time as the water from the chips is incorporated into the oil. For this reason it is best to replace the oil regularly rather than repeatedly reusing it.

Oils that are suitable for high-temperature frying, e.g., deep-frying (above 280°C/500°F) include

- High oleic sunflower or rapeseed oil (not currently readily available on the high street)
- Almond oil
- Peanut oil (marketed as groundnut oil in the UK)
- Soybean oil
- Grapeseed oil.

Oils suitable for medium-temperature frying, e.g. sauces, sautéing, stir-frying; pan fry, baking, salad dressings:

- Rapeseed oil
- Olive oil
- Sesame seed oil
- Sunflower oil.

Unrefined oils, such as virgin olive and rapeseed oils should be restricted to temperatures below 105°C/225°F. They are very delicate and the flavour is lost on heating. They are best used in salad dressings.

Q. *I have recently been diagnosed with high cholesterol, but a friend of mine has been told that she has familial hypercholesterolamia (FH). What is the difference as they both appear to be cholesterol conditions?*

A. High cholesterol can occur as a result of genetic or lifestyle factors, or a combination of both. FH is inherited; it is one of the most common genetic disorders, and it can result in premature heart disease if undiagnosed or not treated. Having FH means that you have high cholesterol from the moment you are conceived. It occurs as a result of a single altered gene passed from parent to child, which influences the cholesterol levels in your blood. This lifelong exposure to high cholesterol is what makes people with FH at high risk of early heart disease. There are other genetic causes of high cholesterol, usually resulting from the small influence of many genes that together raise cholesterol levels. This is called polygenic high cholesterol. People with this form of high cholesterol have a lower risk than those with FH. Both forms of high cholesterol can be affected by your diet and lifestyle.

Q. I have been told I have a cholesterol level of 6.5 mmol/l. Should I try to have a fat-free diet?

A. While it might be sensible to reduce your fat intake, a fat-free or very low-fat diet is not recommended. Instead, reduce your intake of saturated fat and replace it with a combination of unsaturated fats and good-quality complex carbohydrates. This means a bigger emphasis on eating plant (seed and nut) oils and spreads made from these, wholegrains, nuts, seeds, oily fish, fruits, vegetables, and beans, peas and lentils.

A low-fat or a fat-free diet is usually not advised because it lowers your protective HDL cholesterol levels.

Q. I have had a few tests and my high-density lipoprotein (HDL) reading is relatively low. How can I raise my HDL levels?

A. The following lifestyle approach is recommended to raise HDL levels:

• Regular aerobic exercise (any exercise such as walking, jogging, and cycling, etc.) that raises your heart rate for 20–30 minutes at a time.

- Lose weight if overweight by cutting saturated fats and refined carbohydrates (sugary drinks, confectionery, cakes, biscuits, puddings, pies, etc.), watching portion sizes and being more active.
- Eat a Mediterranean type diet
  - Replace saturated fats with unsaturated fats
  - Increase your intake of fruits and vegetables
  - Include oily fish
- Dark chocolate (70 per cent or more in cocoa concentration) is also thought to increase HDL cholesterol level. But it is high in both fat and sugar, so only consume small amounts.
- Stop smoking if you are a smoker.
- Drinking alcohol in small amounts (around one unit or drink a day) may increase HDL levels, but if your triglyceride levels are also high your doctor may advise cutting alcohol out completely.

Q. I have high cholesterol. Should I avoid eating eggs and shellfish?

A. For years, health professionals advised patients to avoid shellfish and eggs because they believed foods high in dietary cholesterol contributed to high blood cholesterol. Recent research has turned this recommendation on its head. Why? Because keeping saturated fat low has been shown to be better at reducing blood cholesterol than restricting eggs and shellfish. So for most people with raised cholesterol the advice is that you do not have to restrict them. However people with an inherited form of high cholesterol such as FH should be more cautious about eating too much of these foods as they can still influence blood cholesterol levels.

Q. My children don't like the taste of fruit and vegetables. How can I incorporate them into my family's diet?

Here are our very best top tips to deal with this common parental concern:

- Children often have to try foods a number of times before they develop a preference for them so it's best to offer a variety of vegetables on a regular basis.
- Don't get upset if they reject them at first. Your aim is to influence their long-term dietary preferences and this can take time.
- Make sure you and your partner provide an excellent role model for eating well.
- Encourage your child to be more engaged by growing their own vegetables and cooking with them.
- Children often eat foods they would not eat at home, such as when at a friend's house, on holiday or even at school, so make the most of these opportunities.
- Try adding vegetables like grated carrot, chopped peppers or sweetcorn to meals like stir-fries, stews and even pizzas.
- Mash vegetables such as swede, parsnips and carrots with potatoes.
- Cutting fruit and vegetables into easy-to-eat sticks often makes them more appealing than a whole piece.
- Don't ask children to eat too much. A portion of fruit and vegetables for a small child is less than that for an adult; a good rule of thumb is the size of the child's fist.
- Make the most of dried fruits, but remember these are sticky and ensure teeth are cleaned regularly.

Q. If something is low in cholesterol, does that mean it's low in fat?

A. Not necessarily. Many foods that are low or free from cholesterol can still be high in fat. Cholesterol is only found in animal foods. Plant-based foods that are high in fat include as nuts, seeds and dark chocolate.

Q. I have been told to avoid taking grapefruit juice since being prescribed a statin. Why is this?

A. Grapefruit contains the compound bergamottin, which interacts with certain enzyme systems in the body, such as cytochrome P-450 and P-glycoprotein. These enzyme systems are responsible for breaking down statins, as well as other drugs, into more manageable chemicals that they can be removed from the body.

When grapefruit juice is consumed, the components in the grapefruit reduce the availability of these enzyme systems, stopping them from breaking down the statin and causing the drug to accumulate in high amounts in the body. This can be dangerous. Not all the statins are affected as some are broken down by different chemical pathways. The main ones that are affected are simvastatin, lovastatin and atorvastatin. Usually a small amount of grapefruit is acceptable but not grapefruit juice because this has a higher concentration of bergamottin. Check the leaflet in the medicines pack if you are in doubt.

Q. I have been diagnosed with high cholesterol. I am a fit woman with a good diet. My question is can taking 1000 mg of cod liver oil capsule per day cause my cholesterol to go up?

A. The effect that 1 g (1000 mg) of any oil/fat would have on your cholesterol has to be negligible. The guideline for women with moderate activity levels is to have no more than 70 g of fat each day of which no more than 20 g should be saturated. A 1 g capsule of cod liver oil is only about 1.5 per cent of your daily fat intake.

There is however a concern with cod liver oil because of its high levels of vitamin A. Vitamin A is a fat-soluble vitamin that is stored in the liver; therefore fish liver is rich in vitamin A. Consuming more than 1500 mcg a day of vitamin A, in the form of retinol, has been associated with bone fractures in women over the age of 50.

The recommended daily intake of vitamin A is 800mcg per day. It is found mainly in full-fat dairy products, liver and oily fish.

Fish oils (as opposed to fish liver oils) do not usually contain vitamin A, but still contain the beneficial long chain omega-3 fatty acids found in cod liver oil, and often in higher amounts.

Q. *I'm scared because I have inherited high cholesterol from my family. How do I cope?*

A. If you think you have inherited high cholesterol then you should discuss this with your GP. If your doctor suspects you have an inherited cholesterol condition such as familial hyper-cholesterolaemia (FH) he should refer you to a lipid clinic where a more formal diagnosis can be made. This involves a fasting blood test, a physical examination and an in-depth discussion around your family's history of heart disease.

It is important to get a diagnosis early because, with effective treatment, people with FH can live a full and healthy life, providing they follow the advice of their doctor. If you are diagnosed as having FH, remember it's just a diagnosis, not a life sentence, and empowers you to make healthy changes to your diet and lifestyle.

Q. *I have familial hypercholesterolaemia (FH) and have been on a cholesterol-lowering diet since the age of 14 and started taking statins at the age of 18. I now have two children aged 2 and 4. At the moment I am giving them full-fat milk to drink. Should I move them on to semi-skimmed milk or are they too young?*

A. It is generally considered that for most children semi-skimmed milk can be introduced from the age of 2 and fully skimmed milk from 5 as part of a balanced overall diet. This, of course, depends on whether your children have healthy appetites and are growing and developing normally. If you are concerned about the saturated fat in whole milk or semi-skimmed milk you could try a 'toddler' milk. Although they have similar energy levels to whole milk they have less saturated fat and contain extra vitamin D and iron, which is lacking in cows' milk.

From the age of 2 years children can now be tested to see if they have inherited the altered gene from the parent who has FH. This would normally be arranged by a lipid clinic, which has facilities for children. Occasionally it is not possible to determine a definitive diagnosis at this age and if this is the case children may need to be monitored and tested at regular intervals.

Q. My doctor has only measured my total cholesterol level. Is this enough, or should I ask for the different levels to be measured?

A. On most occasions it is really helpful to have an indication of the quantity and the quality of cholesterol in your blood. However there are occasions when doctors or clinics might only test the total amount of cholesterol in your blood as part of a screening process. This can be a helpful guide but if the result is high you should have further tests to determine the full profile of blood fats. However, if you are being treated for raised cholesterol, or if you are at high risk of heart disease, your doctor will need a full lipid profile in order to guide him to offer the appropriate therapy.

Q. I am 70 years old and have recently been prescribed a statin. On reading the patient information leaflet (PIL) in my medicine pack I was concerned that it mentions 'taking care if aged over 70'. Why is this, and should I take this medicine?

A. Early trials of statins had fewer patients over the age of 70 so the statement in the PIL reflects this by suggesting caution.

One of the most commonly reported side effects with statins is a generalised muscle pain, a little like the symptoms of flu. Besides muscle and joint pain, older people are more likely to have other medical complaints and be taking a number of other medications. It is this increasing age, other medical problems, and taking a number of medications that can put older people at higher risk of experiencing side effects on statin therapy.

Any side effects you experience when taking a statin have to be balanced against the positive benefits of taking the medicine. It's true that the risk of a heart attack or stroke increases with age but quality of life is also important too. If you do experience any symptoms which you think may be related to your statin, don't ignore them. They are fully and rapidly reversible in the vast majority of cases. It is best not to stop taking the statin before having a frank and open discussion with your GP. They should be able to advise you on the best course of action.

It's important to remember that we all get aches and pains from time to time and it is easy to associate any muscle ache with a medicine you have just started taking. Your doctor is best placed to advise if the symptoms you have are likely to be caused by your treatment.

Q. I have been on a cholesterol-lowering diet and a statin for the last 12 months and after a recent blood test, my doctor told me that I had reached my target levels. What happens now? Can I stop taking the statin?

A. Reaching your cholesterol target is great, but maintaining it is just as important. It is essential that you keep following a healthy diet and lifestyle and keep taking the statin as prescribed. Your doctor will review your progress regularly.

Q. I have high cholesterol but I am underweight too. What foods will help me gain some weight but won't increase my cholesterol levels?

A. If your weight loss has been recent and unintentional, see your doctor to rule out any underlying health problems. If you are consciously restricting your foods because you are worried about increasing your cholesterol levels, here are some tips:

- Keep a food diary so you can review what you routinely eat
- Plan three regular meals plus two or three snacks each day
- Choose a wide variety of foods based on the guidance in this book
- Include good heart-friendly oil-rich foods such as oily fish, nuts, avocado
- Limit food and drinks that fill you up without adding nutrients, such as excess tea and coffee
- Avoid drinking fluids just before and during meals as they may fill you up too quickly
- Have slightly bigger portions or make meals more calorific. For example, have an extra slice of wholegrain toast or spread a generous helping of peanut butter on toast at breakfast or add dried fruit or honey to your breakfast cereal
- Regularly include foods such as unsalted nuts, seeds and dried fruit as snacks
- Use fats high in monounsaturates to make salad dressings and sauté or stir fry your vegetables instead of boiling them
- Cereals, cereal bars, wheatmeal and oatmeal biscuits, and smoothies can be useful as between-meal snacks, but check that they are low in saturated fats i.e. less than 1.5 g saturated fat per 100 g

If you are someone who's always on their feet, set aside time to relax each day!

Gaining weight and keeping it on can be as difficult as losing it and keeping it off. Rather than casually having the occasional extra snack, you may need to work harder to take in more calories than you burn each day.

Q. *If I follow your cholesterol-lowering dietary advice how long should I wait to have a repeat cholesterol test done?*

A. Any effects of diet and lifestyle should be apparent after a few weeks but it is best to wait for at least three months before a repeat cholesterol test for an accurate picture. This three month period is important in helping you to embed diet and lifestyle changes into your daily routine. If you do have a cholesterol test earlier make sure you don't relax your new healthier habits afterwards.

Q. *Is garlic good to help lower cholesterol?*

A. At this time there is not enough evidence to suggest that garlic can lower cholesterol. Sadly many food-based studies are of poor quality and this is the case with garlic and many other food supplements. Nevertheless, together with fresh herbs, garlic is a great way to flavour food without the need to add any salt.

Cutting down on salt, in those with high blood pressure, can help to lower it. A low salt intake can also help prevent high blood pressure in those individuals that are more prone to it. Raised blood pressure is a risk factor for coronary heart disease.

Resources

Alcohol

Alcohol Concern: www.alcoholconcern.org.uk/
Drink Aware: www.drinkaware.co.uk/

Blood pressure

Blood pressure UK: www.bloodpressureuk.org

Diabetes

Diabetes UK: www.diabetes.org.uk/
Diabetes Research and Wellness Foundation: www.drwf.org.uk/

Exercise

Keep Fit Association: www.keepfit.org.uk/
Ramblers Association: www.ramblers.org.uk/
Sport England: www.sportengland.org/

General

NHS Livewell: www.nhs.uk/livewell
Change for Life: www.nhs.uk/change4life/
NHS Choices: www.nhs.uk/Pages/HomePage.aspx
Patient Opinion: www.patientopinion.org.uk
Patient UK: www.patient.co.uk/

Healthy eating

British Dietetic Association Factsheets: www.bda.uk.com/
    foodfacts/home
British Nutrition Foundation: www.nutrition.org.uk/
Ultimate Cholesterol Lowering Diet: www.heartuk.org.uk/UCLP

HEART

British Cardiac Patients Association: www.bcpa.co.uk/
HEART UK—The Cholesterol Charity: www.heartuk.org.uk
Sudden Arrhythmia Death Syndromes: www.sads.org/
British Heart Foundation: www.bhf.org.uk/

Medicines

Your statin: www.mystatinstatus.co.uk/
Electronic medicines compendium: www.medicines.org.uk/emc/
X-Pil: www.xpil.medicines.org.uk/

Smoking

ASH: www.ash.org.uk/
NHS Smoke Free: www.nhs.uk/smokefree

Stress

Anxiety UK: www.anxietyuk.org.uk/
Work-related Stress: http://www.hse.gov.uk/stress/
Samaritans: www.samaritans.org/

Stroke

The Stroke Association: www.stroke.org.uk/

Weight

My Healthy Waist: www.myhealthywaist.org/welcome/index.html
Teen Weight Wise: www.teenweightwise.com
Weight Wise: www.bdaweightwise.com

Index